BEER, WINE, OR VODKA?

WHAT SHOULD I DRINK AND HOW MUCH FOR BETTER HEALTH?

AMITAVA DASGUPTA, Ph.D.

Published by KHARIS PUBLISHING, imprint of
KHARIS MEDIA LLC

Copyright © 2016 Amitava Dasgupta

ISBN-13: 978-1-946277-05-3
ISBN-10: 1-946277-05-3

All KHARIS PUBLISHING products are available at special
quantity discounts for bulk purchase for sales promotions,
premiums, fund-raising, and educational needs. For details, write:

Kharis Publishing
709 SW Elmside Drive
Bentonville,
AR 72712
Tel: 1-479-903-8160
info@kharispublishing.com
www.kharispublishing.com

CONTENTS

PREFACE

Approximately 60% of all Americans consume alcohol; it is important to note that drinking in moderation has many health benefits including a lower risk of cardiovascular diseases (heart and coronary artery diseases), stroke, type 2 diabetes, and rheumatoid arthritis. Both beer and wine contain many beneficial organic compounds (polyphenols) which are not only antioxidants, but some of these compounds also have anticancer properties. However, there are controversies regarding the moderate consumption of alcohol and breast cancer in women. This book is a consumer health book written with the goal of empowering people with current scientific knowledge related to the health benefits of the low to moderate consumption of alcohol and also to counteract some popular health beliefs, for example, that drinking alcohol during breastfeeding is a good practice because it increases breast milk secretion, that drinking beer before exercising is a good idea, that drinking beer is associated with weight gain, and that drinking red wine is far better than drinking white wine or beer. Scientific evidence does not support these popular beliefs and my goal is to educate readers with the latest scientific data, presented in simple language without medical and scientific jargon.

Drinking and driving is a major issue. How much alcohol consumption is safe before driving? What is the relationship between blood alcohol and the number of alcoholic drinks consumed based on gender and body weight? Usually the Widmark formula is used for calculating blood alcohol levels from the number of drinks consumed, from body weight, and from gender as well as from the time frame involved in consuming these alcoholic drinks. This is possible because all alcoholic beverages contain approximately 14 gm of absolute alcohol (chapter 1). The guidelines for safe drinking and driving is discussed in detail in Chapter 2. Moreover, the technology used for breath alcohol and blood alcohol measurement is also discussed. In general, blood alcohol measured in crime or forensic laboratories using headspace gas chromatography, is the gold standard. Although results from evidentiary Breathalyzers are acceptable in courts as evidence, Breathalyzers are subjected to interferences. This issue is discussed in detail in chapter 2 with tips about what to do if a person is stopped by a police officer with a suspected DWI. Many health benefits of drinking in moderation are discussed in detail in chapter 3.

However, heavy drinking is associated with health hazards which are addressed in chapter 4. Heavy drinking is associated with a fatty liver, while alcoholism may cause cirrhosis of the liver, a potentially fatal disease. In general, women are more susceptible to adverse effects of excessive drinking than men. Underage drinking is a huge problem. Since the brain of an adolescent is still developing, underage drinking may have adverse effects on their brain. Girls are more affected than boys. However, many environmental factors are associated with underage drinking. These factors are addressed in chapter 5. Although offspring of alcoholics have 4 to 10 times higher risks of abusing alcohol in adulthood than offspring of nonalcoholic parents, there is no single gene which is associated with alcoholism. Genetic factors contributing to the overall susceptibility of alcohol abuse, may contribute 50%, while environmental factors may contribute 50%. Many positive environmental factors have protective effects on alcohol abuse. Therefore, it is absolutely possible for an offspring of alcoholic parents to be a teetotaler. Moreover, alcohol abuse and alcoholism are psychiatric illnesses which can be cured by proper treatment. If you know someone or have a loved one with alcohol problems advise them to seek medical help as soon as possible. In chapter 6, I discuss what should be your favorite drink: beer, wine, or vodka (liquor).

I would like to thank my wife, Alice, for her support during my long evening and weekend hours I devoted to write this book. If readers enjoy this book, my efforts will be rewarded.

Respectfully Submitted by

Amitava Dasgupta, Ph.D., DABCC
Houston

1 ALL ALCOHOLIC DRINKS CONTAIN THE SAME AMOUNT OF ALCOHOL

Introduction

Fermentation of sugar by yeast produces a colorless liquid known as ethyl alcohol or simply alcohol. A very small amount of alcohol is also produced endogenously due to normal metabolism, but such a level is so low that it cannot be detected during routine blood alcohol measurement. Drinking alcoholic beverages is a common practice in the United States and in many other countries worldwide.

Drinking alcoholic beverages in moderation (up to 2 drinks a day for males and up to 1 drink per day for females) has many health benefits, but heavy alcohol consumption is hazardous to our health. According to the 2014 National Survey on Drug Use and Health conducted by the Substance Abuse and Mental Health Administration (SAMHA), a U.S. government agency, 139.7 million Americans consumed alcohol during the past 30 days, including 16.3 million Americans who were heavy alcohol users (drinking 5 or more drinks on 1occasion on 5or more days in the past 30 days). It was also estimated that 60.9 million Americans were binge drinkers. In general, more males abused alcohol than females.

The World Health Organization (WHO) estimated that the 5.1% global burden of disease and injuries are related to alcohol abuse (1). Heavy consumption of alcohol is associated with domestic violence, decreased productivity, increased risk of motor vehicle accidents, job-related injuries, and an increased risk of liver disease, stroke, and cancer. Alcohol is involved in many fatal car accidents and according to the National Highway Traffic Safety Administration, approximately 30% of traffic fatalities are linked to excessive alcohol consumption, which is also responsible for 10-18% of injured patients who are admitted to hospital emergency rooms in the United States. Moreover, the economic cost of excessive alcohol consumption was estimated to be $223.5 billion annually in the United States (2).

Why Do People Drink?

Professor Robert Dudley (2004) of the University of California, Berkeley, posed a rational for why people drink in his "Drunken Monkey Hypothesis." Primates, our ancestors several million years ago, used fruits as their major source of diet. Those capable of detecting the smell of alcohol in ripe fruits (while fruit is being ripened, alcohol is produced from sugar by yeast present on the fruit skin), survived better due to natural selection. As a result, when humans evolved from primates one to two million years ago, a keen taste for alcohol probably became a part of the genetic makeup. Interestingly, even today, most people consume alcohol during evening meals (3).

History of Drinking

The first historical evidence of alcoholic beverages came from the archaeological discovery of Stone Age beer jugs which dated approximately 10,000 years ago. Egyptians probably consumed wine and beer approximately 6,000 years ago. The earliest evidence of alcohol use in China dated back to 5000 BC, when alcohol was mainly produced from rice, honey, and fruits. In ancient India, alcohol beverages were called "sura" and the use of such drinks was documented in ancient Ayurvedic texts written between 3000 and 2000 BC. Ancient Ayurvedic texts also warned against the abuse of alcohol, calling it a poison at higher dosages. Beer was known to Babylonians as early as 2700 BC. In ancient Greece, wine making was common practice in 1700 BC. Hippocrates identified numerous medicinal properties of wine but was critical of drunkenness (4).

In ancient civilizations, alcohol was used primarily to quench thirst because water was contaminated with bacteria. Beer was a drink for common people, while wine was the preferred drink for elites. In ancient Eastern civilization, drinking alcoholic beverages for thirst quenching was less common because drinking tea was very popular in Asian countries. During the boiling process to prepare tea, all pathogens died, thus making tea drinking a safe healthy practice.

Yeast can produce alcoholic beverages containing up to 15% alcohol; at that alcohol concentration yeast cells can no longer survive. In order to prepare alcoholic beverages with a much higher alcohol content, distillation techniques are needed. Distillation methods were well recognized in Europe probably around the eleventh century. In 1791, however, a tax was introduced, known as the "Whiskey tax" on both privately and publicly brewed distilled whiskey. The Whiskey tax was repealed by President Thomas Jefferson in 1802, but a new alcohol tax was temporarily imposed between 1814 and 1817, to pay for the War of 1812. In 1862, President Abraham Lincoln introduced an alcohol tax to pay for the costs of the Civil War. The act also created the office of Internal Revenue. In 1920, alcohol was prohibited in the United States but Congress repealed the law in 1933. In 1978, President Jimmy Carter signed a bill to legalize the home brewing of beer for personal use for the first time since Prohibition (5).

How Are Alcoholic Beverages Produced?

All alcoholic beverages are produced by a process known as "fermentation" where yeast converts simple sugars (fructose and glucose) under anaerobic conditions (absence of oxygen) into ethyl alcohol (alcohol) and into carbon dioxide. Fructose is the sugar present in many fruits and vegetables. Louis Pastor first scientifically described the fermentation process. Yeasts are classified as fungus and over 1,500 different species are found in nature. Usually, yeast known as *Saccharomyces cerevisiae*, is used for baking and fermenting while *Candida* causes yeast infections in humans.

In the first step of producing beer, barley is soaked in hot water allowing malt to germinate, thus releasing amylases (malting process), enzymes needed for converting starch (carbohydrate) present in grains into sugars. Different roasting times and temperatures produce different colors of malt from the same grain; the darker the malt, the darker the beer. Although barley is the main grain used for brewing beer, other sources of starch such as rye, wheat, and even rice may also be used. After the malting process, the malt is again soaked in hot water for an hour and then the liquid, which mostly contains sugar, is separated from grain. The extract (wort) is boiled to ensure sterility and then hops are added for obtaining the characteristic bitter taste of the beer. Finally, the liquid is cooled and yeast is added for fermentation. Most beers are produced using "bottom-fermenting yeast" and the brewing process is conducted at low temperatures (50 to 64^{0}F). In this case, after fermentation yeast cells settle at the bottom, a small amount of foam is produced. Brewing using "top-fermenting yeasts" requires higher temperatures (61 to 75^{0}F). After fermentation, yeast cells float at the top of the liquid and foam (due to carbon dioxide) is also produced. This type of fermentation is used to produce "ale types of beer" with higher alcohol contents (fruiter, sweeter beers).

Usually wines are made from harvesting ripe grapes in a vineyard. The first step is to produce a must from crushed grapes which may contain grape juice, seeds, and skin. During the production of white wine, grape skins are removed but in red wine, grape skins are included. Red wine is fermented at a higher temperature (up to 85^{0}F) than white wine (64 to 68^{0}F). After fermentation, solid residues are allowed to settle and wine is placed in a new container such as a wooden oak barrel for aging. The characteristic flavor of wine is generated during the aging process due to complex chemical reactions. Commercial brewers have strict quality control procedures in each step of wine manufacturing to ensure the high quality of the end product. Acidity and the specific gravity of wine is carefully controlled to meet their specifications. The aroma of wine is due to 600 to 800 volatile compounds mostly characteristic of grapes used for wine production. Usually, residual carbon dioxide is not allowed to stay in wine. However, Champagne is supplemented with carbon dioxide in order to achieve its bubbly appearance. Carbon dioxide is also added to produce sparkling wine. In port wine, additional alcohol is added after production in order to increase its alcoholic content.

Alcoholic beverages produced by fermentation and distillation are known as spirits. After fermentation, the alcohol content is usually 14-16%, but in order to make alcoholic beverages with 40% alcohol, a process known as distillation is used. When alcohol and a water mixture is boiled, alcohol starts evaporating at 78^{0}C and the vapor is mostly composed of alcohol. Then the vapor is allowed to pass through a tube (condenser) which is cooled and alcohol vapor is converted into liquid again. This process is called distillation and the instrument that is utilized is called a still. However, many beneficial organic compounds present in beer and in wine are not present in liquors because such compounds are lost during the distillation process. In addition, no carbohydrate is present in liquors. However, when liquor is aged using a wooden barrel, some beneficial organic compounds present in the wood may leak into the liquor. Starting materials for preparing various types of alcoholic beverages are listed in table 1.

Table 1. Fermenting material for producing beer, wine, and liquors

Alcoholic beverage	Fermented from
Beer	Barley (most common) but rye may also be used
Sake (Japanese beer)	Rice
White wine	Grapes without grape skin
Red wine	Grapes with grape skin
Plum wine	Plums
Hard cider (apple cider)	Apples
Brandy/cognac (distilled wine)	Grapes
Bourbon, whiskey	Corn
Scotch whiskey, Irish whiskey, etc.	Barley
Vodka	Originally made from potatoes but now wheat is a popular ingredient. Rye or corn can be also used.
Gin	Juniper berry
Rum	Sugarcane, molasses, or sugarcane juice
Tequila	Made from blue agave plant found in the surroundings of the city of Tequila, Mexico

All Alcoholic Beverages Contain 14 gm of Alcohol

In the United States, a standard drink is defined as a bottle of beer (12 fl oz, 355 mL) containing 5% alcohol, 8.5 fl oz of malt liquor containing 7% alcohol, a 5-fl oz glass of wine containing 12% alcohol, 3.5 fl oz of fortified wine like sherry or port containing about 17% alcohol, 2-3 fl oz of cordial or liqueur containing 24% alcohol, or one shot of a distilled spirits such as gin, rum, vodka, or whiskey (1.5 fl oz). Therefore, a bottle of beer contains 12 fl oz of beer multiplied by 0.05 representing 5% alcohol content to calculate the total amount of alcohol, or 0.6 fl oz of absolute alcohol. For calculating the alcohol content in grams, a bottle of beer contains 355 mL of alcohol which must be multiplied by 0.05 (5 % alcohol content) and 0.789 (density of alcohol 0.789 gm/mL) which yields 14 gm. Similarly, using this formula, it can be shown that a standard alcoholic beverage contains approximately 14 gm of alcohol. However, a bottle of light beer (4.2% alcohol) contains 0.5 fl oz of alcohol (11.8 gm alcohol). Therefore, consuming one bottle of light beer is equivalent to 0.8 standard drinks (table 2).

Table 2. Alcohol content of various drinks

Alcoholic beverage	Approximate alcohol content	Serving size	Approximate amount of total alcohol
Standard beer	5 %	12 fl oz (355 mL)	0.6 oz/14 gm
Malt liquor	7%	8.5 fl oz (251 mL)	0.59 oz/13.9 gm
Table wine	12%	5 fl oz (148 mL)	0.6 oz/14 gm
Fortified wine	17%	3.5 fl oz (104 ml)	0.59 oz/13.9 gm
Cordial or liqueur containing	24%	2-3 fl oz (59-88 mL)	0.48-0.72 oz/ 11.2-16.7 gm
Brandy or cognac	40%	1.5 fl oz (44 mL)	0.6 oz/14 gm

80 Proof distilled spirit (vodka, whiskey, rum, or tequila)	40%	1.5 fl oz (44 mL)	0.6 oz/14 gm
Scotch, whiskey	55-60%	1.5 fl oz (44 mL)	0.83-0.9 oz/ 19.0-20.8 gm

Important conversion factor: 1 fl oz = 29.57 mL

Density of alcohol = 0.789 gm/mL (alcohol is lighter than water; water has a density of 1.00 gm/mL

The major advantage of knowing that a standard drink contains 14 gm of alcohol concerns the calculation of blood alcohol based on the number of drinks consumed by an individual, the time period of consuming all such alcohol beverages, the gender of the individual, and body weight. A commonly used formula for calculating blood alcohol is the Widmark formula. This formula is often used by toxicologists during criminal prosecutions involving alcohol-related cases. A toxicologist may want to know if the blood alcohol determined in the laboratory of an individual accused of driving with impairment (DWI) is consistent with their alleged drinking history. (see chapter 2 for more details).

The alcoholic content of various drinks is often expressed as *proof,* a term originated in the eighteenth century when British sailors were paid with money as well as with rum. In order to ensure that the rum was not diluted with water, it was "proofed" by dousing gunpowder with it and setting it on fire. If the gunpowder failed to ignite, it indicated that rum was diluted with excess water. A sample of rum which was 100 proof contained approximately 57% alcohol by volume. In the United States, proof to alcohol by volume is defined as a ratio of 1:2. Therefore, beer, which has 5% alcohol by volume, is defined as 10 proof. In general, multiplying the alcohol content of a drink by a factor of 2, produces the "proof" of alcohol. Currently, in the United States, the alcohol content of a drink is measured by the percentage of alcohol by volume. The Code of Federal Regulations requires that the label of alcoholic beverages must state the alcohol content by volume. The regulation permits, but does not require, the "proof" of the drink to be printed.

Alcoholic beverages such as beer and wine consist of water, alcohol, and variable amounts of carbohydrates (very small amounts of residual sugar and starch left after fermentation). However, distilled liquors such as cognac, vodka, whiskey, and rum contain no carbohydrates. Therefore, any calories derived from drinking alcoholic beverages come mostly from the alcohol content and from some from carbohydrate and residual sugar present in the drink. In general, 14 gm of alcohol, which is present in 1 standard drink, produces 98 calories. However, drinking an alcoholic beverage may produce more calories due to the presence of residual carbohydrates. Alcoholic fruit drinks, for example, Pina colada, contains 490 calories. The calorie content of various alcoholic beverages is given in table 3.

Table 3. Average calories associated with various alcoholic beverages

Alcoholic beverage	Average serving size	Average calorie content of the drink
Regular beer	12 fl oz	153
Light beer	12 fl oz	103
Red wine	5 fl oz	125
White wine	5 fl oz	121
Sweet wine	3.5 fl oz	165
Champagne	4 fl oz	84
Vermouth sweet	3 fl oz	140
Vermouth dry	3 fl oz	105
Gin, rum, vodka, whiskey, or tequila	1.5 fl oz	97
Brandy, or cognac	1.5 fl oz	98
Pina colada	9 fl oz	490

Source of information: National Institute on Alcohol Abuse and Alcoholism, National Institute of Health website:

http://rethinkingdrink.niaaa.nih.gov/tools/calculators/calorie-calculator.aspx

Drinking Patterns in the United States

According to a Gallup poll conducted in 2013, 60% of Americans reported drinking alcoholic beverages and among them, 36 % respondents preferred drinking beer, 35% wine, and 23% liquor. However, according to a 1992 survey, 47% preferred drinking beer compared to only 27% who preferred wine, indicating that wine drinking is gaining popularity in the United States among people who consume alcohol. Interestingly, drinking beer, according to the poll, was most popular among young people 18-29 years of age, where 41% preferred beer in a 2013 survey (down from 71% in a 1992-1994 survey) as well as among 30-49-year-olds (43% preferred beer in a 2012-2013 survey, down from 48% in a 1992-1994 survey). However, drinking wine was most popular among people over 50 years of age (in a 2013 poll, 46 % preferred drinking wine, compared to 29% who preferred drinking beer). Drinking wine was also more popular among women (52% preferred wine, 24% liquor, and 20% beer while 53% of men preferred drinking beer, 22% liquor, and 20% wine) (6).

Effect of Alcohol on Nutrition

Most people in the United States consume alcohol moderately and as a result approximately 4.5% of their total daily calories are coming from alcohol, but for people consuming more alcohol, up to 10% of all of their calories may derive from alcohol. In contrast, alcoholics may derive half of all their calories from drinking. The majority of people who consume alcohol moderately, usually show insignificant or no detectable nutritional impairment. However, excess alcohol consumption may interfere with the breakdown of food by inhibiting the secretion of digestive enzymes from the pancreas. Moreover, excess alcohol consumption may also impair the absorption of nutrients including vitamins from the stomach and from the intestine. Alcoholics may suffer from a deficiency of vitamins including vitamin D, which is associated with reduced bone density, thus increasing the risk of fractures. In addition, a deficiency of minerals such as calcium magnesium, iron, and zinc, are also common among alcoholics (7). Another study reported that chronic alcoholic patients are frequently deficient in folate, vitamin A, thiamine (vitamin B1), and vitamin B6. Although inadequate dietary intake is one of the factors causing such a deficiency, other factors such as reduced absorption of these vitamins from food and altered storage may also be responsible (8). Thiamine deficiency is responsible for alcohol-induced brain damage including Wernicke-Korsakoff syndrome which is mainly observed in chronic alcoholics (see chapter 4). Gloria et al. (1997) reported that 18.1% of chronic alcoholic patients they studied were malnourished (9).

Conclusions

Although most Americans who consume alcohol are moderate drinkers, an estimated 16.3 million are heavy drinkers. There are many health benefits of drinking in moderation including a reduced risk of cardiovascular diseases , reduced risk of stroke, and increased longevity. Although moderate drinkers derive these health benefits, with heavy alcohol consumption, all of these health benefits disappear. In addition, alcoholism is also associated with many health hazards including cirrhosis of the liver, which may be a potentially fatal disease.

2 GUIDELINES FOR DRINKING IN MODERATION AND AVOIDING DWI

Introduction

Drinking in moderation has many health benefits. If an individual follows the guidelines for drinking in moderation and consumes alcoholic beverages with food, there is absolutely no risk of being charged with Driving with Impairment or Driving while Impaired or Driving while Intoxicated (DWI) or with Driving under the Influence (DUI). Although DWI and DUI are similar terms, in some states, DUI is considered as a lesser crime than DWI, but in other states there may not be any distinction. Although alcohol is a common factor in both DWI and DUI cases, impairment may also be caused if a person is driving under the influence of an illicit drug or even under the influence of prescription pain management opioid drugs such as oxycodone, oxymorphone, hydrocodone, hydromorphone, codeine, morphine, or tramadol as well as benzodiazepine drugs (used for treating insomnia or anxiety) such as alprazolam, clonazepam, diazepam, lorazepam, or temazepam.

In all states, the legal limit of driving is 0.08% whole

blood alcohol (80 mg in 100 milliliters of blood, which is expressed as mg/dL) in a person 21 years of age or older (the legal drinking age in the U.S.). If an individual is younger than 21 and has a blood alcohol significantly lower than 0.08%, in many states with "zero tolerance policy" they may be charged with DWI or DUI. Depending on the level of blood alcohol (usually 0.08% or higher but less than 0.12%), in some states, a person may take advantage of plea bargaining and may face probation if no one is injured. However, for second or third offenses, jail time, suspension of drivers' licenses, and fines may result if convicted with DWI or DUI. If someone is seriously injured or killed as a result of drunk driving, the penalty may be significant even for the first offense. Therefore, the best practice is to drink sensibly, thus avoiding a DWI or DUI charge.

Physiological Effects of Alcohol

Substantial research has established that the effect of alcohol on the brain depends on the blood alcohol level. Even just after consuming from 1/2 to 1 drink (depending on gender and body weight), the blood alcohol level may reach 0.03% and at that level a person feels the pleasurable effects of alcohol including mild euphoria, happiness, less shyness, and more social interactions. Although such pleasurable effects of alcohol may continue with blood alcohol levels of up to 0.05 %, some impairment of motor skills may be observed even at that blood level.

The legal limit of driving in all states in the United States is 0.08% in whole blood which is generous because in many European countries, the legal limit is 0.05% or even less. At a blood alcohol level above 0.08%, a significant impairment of motor skills is observed. At a blood alcohol level of 0.3% and higher, a complete loss of consciousness and even death may occur. Celik et al. (2013) reported that postmortem blood alcohol levels ranged from 136 to 608 mg/dL (0.136% to 0.608%) in 39 individuals who died due to alcohol overdoses. Most of these deceased were male (1).

Death from alcohol poisoning is usually attributed to paralysis of the respiratory and circulatory centers in the brain causing asphyxiation (impairment of breathing).

Guidelines for Drinking in Moderation

The U.S. Department of Agriculture (USDA) and the U.S. Department of Health and Human Services (USDHHS) jointly publish "Dietary Guidelines for Americans" every five years, suggesting to Americans what constitutes a balanced diet. These guidelines also include suggestions for drinking in moderation. It is important to note that alcohol is not a component USDA food pattern. If alcohol is consumed, the calories from alcohol must be accounted for when other foods are consumed so that the daily calorie intake does not exceed the recommended limit (1,600-2,400 calories per day for women, and 2,000-3,000 calories per day for men). The latest Dietary Guidelines for Americans, 2015 to 2020, suggested that if alcohol is consumed it should be consumed in moderation following these guidelines:

•Recommended Consumption: Up to 1 drink per day for women, and up to 2drinks per day for men-- and only by adults of legal drinking age.

One drink is defined as containing 14 gm (0.6 fl oz) of alcohol. One alcoholic drink is equivalent to drinking 12 fl oz of regular beer (5% alcohol), 5 fl oz of wine (12% alcohol), or 1.5 fl oz of 80 proof distilled spirits (40% alcohol). If light beer is consumed (4.2% alcohol) it should be considered as 0.8 drink. Mixed drinks (including fruit drinks mixed with sprits) with more than 1.5 fl oz of alcohol should be considered as more than 1 drink. The formula for calculating drink equivalents is as follows:

Drink equivalent = Volume of alcoholic beverage x alcohol content/0.6

For example, drinking 16 fl oz of beer containing 5% alcohol is equivalent to 1.33 drinks.

The Federal Food and Drug Administration (FDA) has determined that mixing alcohol and caffeine is not a safe practice and recommended four manufacturers of alcoholic beverages containing caffeine to discontinue the use of caffeine in alcoholic drinks. People who mix alcohol and caffeine may drink more alcohol and become more intoxicated than they realize, increasing the risk of alcohol-related adverse events.

Excessive alcohol consumption includes both heavy drinking and binge drinking. Heavy drinking is defined as consuming 8 or more drinks by a woman, or 15 or more drinks by a man in one week. In the United States, approximately 50% of adults consume alcohol on a regular basis, while another 14% are infrequent drinkers. An estimated 9% of men consume more than 2drinks per day and an estimated 4% of women consume more than 1 drink per day.

Binge drinking (consuming 5 or more drinks in one sitting by males, or 4 or more drinks by a female at least once a month) is also associated with many risks and produces blood alcohol 0.08% or above. The Substance Abuse and Mental Health Services Administration (SAMHSA), an agency of the National Institute of Health, develops guidelines for workplace alcohol and drug testing for federal employees; this agency has slightly different guidelines for binge drinking (see chapter 4).

One obvious risk of binge drinking is the possibility of being charged with DWI if stopped by the police because binge drinking always produces a blood alcohol level over the legal limit of driving. Binge drinking is a serious public health issue not only for high school or college students, but for people of any age. Statistics from the Center for Disease Control and Prevention (CDC) indicates that 16.6% of U.S. adults are involved in binge drinking approximately four times a month, consuming approximately 8 drinks per binge session. Binge drinking is also more common among young adults aged 18-34 and among people with household incomes of $75,000 or more per year than among people with lower incomes. Moreover, binge drinking is more common in men than in women.

Binge drinking is responsible for over 50% of 80,000 annual deaths caused by alcohol each year in the United States. A study found that 39% of full-time college students (ages 18-22) had been binge drinking at least on one occasion in the past 30 days. Full-time college students were also involved in significantly more episodes of binge drinking than their counterparts not attending college but belonging to the same age group. The authors commented that binge drinking is a leading culprit of preventable deaths on college campuses (2).

Energy drinks are gaining popularity among young adults as well as among underage drinkers. Studies have indicated that energy drinks may increase the craving for alcohol and for binge drinking. When an energy drink, which often contains caffeine, is combined with alcohol, the desire to drink alcohol is more pronounced compared to drinking alcohol without the consumption of an energy drink. Moreover, the pleasurable experience of drinking alcohol is also enhanced by consuming energy drinks (3). Important facts regarding binge drinking are listed in table 1.

Table 1. Important facts about binge drinking

•Binge drinking is more common among college students and among the young adult age group, 18-34.

•Binge drinking always produces blood alcohol above the legal limit of driving (0.08% in whole blood).

•Binge drinking is a leading culprit of preventable deaths on college campuses.

•People with an annual income of $75,000 or more are more likely to engage in binge drinking than   people with a lower-income group.

•More men than women participate in binge drinking.

•Consumption of energy drinks may increase the risk of consuming more alcohol and binge drinking.

Pregnant women should not drink alcohol at all to avoid any potential ill effects of alcohol on the fetus (explained later in the chapter). In addition, alcohol should not be consumed if an individual is taking certain medications. Usually, labeling of such medication clearly warns against drinking. Moreover, certain people who cannot control their impulses during drinking should avoid drinking altogether. People who should not drink at all are listed in table 2.

Table 2. When not to drink at all

When not to drink	Reason
Pregnant woman	Alcohol crosses the placenta and causes harm to the fetus. This includes birth defects, miscarriage, stillbirth, and premature birth.
Women who are breastfeeding	Alcohol is present in the breast milk and may discourage a newborn from drinking breast milk.
When taking certain medications	Certain antibiotics and other medications interact with alcohol, causing toxicity. These medications also include some over-the-counter medications (especially cold medications).
Individuals who have problems with impulse control	Some people cannot control their drinking behavior and they should avoid drinking.
People who do not drink due to religious reasons or for other reasons	Approximately 40% of Americans are teetotalers for a variety of reasons. Current guidelines discourage these individuals to start drinking in moderation for health reasons.

Studies have shown that peer pressure affects drinking patterns especially underage drinking. If young adults are associated with non-drinking friends and peers or living with roommates who do not drink, it reduces the risk of underage drinking. Relationships with parents and their attitudes toward alcohol consumption may also affect underage drinking patterns (see chapter 5).

Why Is the Legal Age of Drinking 21?

The minimum legal age of drinking in the United States is 21. The current law for the minimum legal age of drinking has been in effect since July 1988, in all 50 states and in the District of Columbia. This law is not intended to punish young adults but is based on sound scientific research. Surveys tracking alcohol consumption among high school students and among young adults demonstrated that drinking declined since the late 1970s, but most of the decline occurred early in the 1990s, when states adopted the minimum legal age of drinking at 21 years of age. Among fatally injured drivers ages 16-20, the percentage with positive blood alcohol (alcohol level at or higher than the legal limit) declined from 61% in 1982, to 31% in 1995. Moreover, studies have shown that adopting the minimum legal age of drinking at 21 years results in the reduction in problematic drinking, drinking and driving, and alcohol-related accidents among young people (4). The law regarding the minimum legal age of drinking has clearly reduced alcohol consumption and its potential harm to young adults. Carpenter and Dobkin (2011) estimated that if the drinking age was lowered to 18 years, there would be an additional 8 deaths per 100,000 people per year in the 18-20 age groups due to alcohol-related fatalities (5).

The human brain is still developing at the age of 18, which is often referred to as adulthood. Neurobiological research indicates that the final stage of maturation of the human brain may continue during the ages of 18-24, which is considered as emerging adulthood. There are neurobiological consequences of underage drinking because alcohol may impair the final stage of maturational refinement of the human brain. Discouraging alcohol consumption until neurobiological adulthood is reached is important in minimizing alcohol-related disruption in the brain development and in the decision-making capacity as well as for reducing the negative behavioral consequences associated with underage drinking (6).

Always Drink Alcohol with Food

When alcohol is consumed, about 20% is absorbed from the stomach and the rest is absorbed from the small intestine by passive diffusion. The highest blood alcohol concentration (peak) is usually observed between 30 and 60 minutes after alcohol consumption. No one should drink on an empty stomach because higher peak blood alcohol will be observed due to the higher absorption of alcohol from the empty stomach. Food substantially slows down the absorption of alcohol and sipping alcohol instead of drinking also slows the absorption of alcohol from the gastrointestinal tract. The presence of food in the stomach before consuming alcohol delays gastric emptying and reduces the rate of delivery of alcohol in the duodenum, thus lowering the alcohol absorption rate.

The effect of food on the absorption and metabolism of alcohol has been studied extensively in the past. In one study, ten healthy male volunteers consumed a moderate dosage of alcohol in the morning after an overnight fast or immediately after breakfast (two cheese sandwiches, one boiled egg, orange juice, and fruit yogurt). Subjects who consumed alcohol on an empty stomach felt more intoxicated than the subjects who consumed the same amount of alcohol after breakfast. The blood alcohol analysis revealed that the average peak blood alcohol in subjects who consumed alcohol on an empty stomach was 104 mg/dL. In contrast, the average peak blood alcohol in subjects who consumed alcohol after eating breakfast was 67 mg/dL. Moreover, the metabolism of alcohol was also more rapid in volunteers who consumed alcohol after breakfast compared to volunteers who consumed alcohol on an empty stomach. The authors concluded that food in the stomach before drinking not only reduced the peak blood alcohol concentration, but also increased the elimination of alcohol from the body (7). Interestingly, any food can slow down the absorption of alcohol from the stomach; it does not need to be a special kind of food, for example, protein or carbohydrate. Therefore, it is recommended that drinkers:

• Consume alcohol with food.
• Sip rather than drink alcohol.

How the Body Eliminates Alcohol

After drinking, alcohol dehydrogenase present in gastric mucosa metabolizes a part of alcohol before it is absorbed. After alcohol is absorbed, it is eliminated from the circulation, first by the action of alcohol dehydrogenase which is also present in the liver, and then by the action of another enzyme, aldehyde dehydrogenase, which is also present in the liver. The final product is acetate, which breaks down into carbon dioxide and water; this is responsible for getting calories from alcohol.

Ethyl alcohol (alcohol) $\xrightarrow{\text{ADH}}$ Acetaldehyde $\xrightarrow{\text{ALDH}}$ Acetate
ADH: Alcohol dehydrogenase enzyme, ALDH: Aldehyde dehydrogenase enzyme

In alcoholics, another liver enzyme known as CYP2E1 can also convert alcohol into acetaldehyde. This enzymatic pathway is activated when the alcohol dehydrogenase enzyme is saturated due to excessive blood alcohol levels. Another enzyme, catalase, can also convert alcohol into acetaldehyde but this pathway is a minor pathway for alcohol metabolism. Regardless of pathways by which acetaldehyde is formed, it is finally converted into acetate by the action of the aldehyde dehydrogenase enzyme. Another minor pathway of alcohol metabolism is to undergo conjugation with other molecules by the action of specific liver enzymes forming ethyl glucuronide and ethyl sulfate. These molecules are used as alcohol biomarkers.

The metabolism of alcohol follows zero order kinetics which means regardless of the amount of alcohol present in the blood, only a fixed part of alcohol is eliminated per hour. In contrast, for many medications, the higher the level of medication in the blood, the faster is the elimination. This process is called first-order kinetics. After drinking alcohol on an empty stomach elimination of alcohol from the body is usually 10-15 mg/dL per hour regardless of initial alcohol concentration in the blood. However, if alcohol is consumed after eating a meal the rate of elimination is usually higher (15-20 mg/dL per hour). Alcoholics may metabolize alcohol at a much higher rate with an elimination rate of 25-35 mg/dL per hour due to activation of CYP2E1 pathway. In general, it can be assumed that in moderate drinkers, the average elimination rate of alcohol is 15 mg/dL per hour (reduction of blood alcohol level by 0.015% whole blood per hour) (8). For example, if a male with a body weight of 150 pounds consumes 5 drinks in one hour, his estimated blood alcohol should be around 150 mg/dL (0.15%). His blood alcohol concentration should decrease by 0.015% per hour and it will take approximately 4.7 hours for blood alcohol to reach 0.08%.

Why Women Should Drink Less than Men

The guidelines for moderate drinking recommend that women consume less alcohol than men. The main reason is that the water content of the human body is gender specific. In general, a woman has lesser amount of body water (52% average) compared to men (61% average). As a result, after drinking the same amount of alcohol, a man usually has a lower peak blood alcohol level compared to a woman with the same body weight because less body water is available in a woman to dissolve the same amount of alcohol compared to a man. Marshall et al. (1983), using 9 normal women and 10 normal men, observed that after ingestion of the same amount of alcohol (0.5 gm/per kg bodyweight), women showed higher peak blood alcohol levels than men (mean: 88 mg/dL in women and mean: 75 mg/dL in men) (9). In general, after consuming the same amount of alcohol (based on body weight), a woman appears to become more impaired than a man.

After consuming alcohol, a small amount is metabolized by alcohol dehydrogenase present in gut mucosa and the rate of first pass metabolism of alcohol is slightly higher in men than in women. Moreover, after absorption from the gastrointestinal tract, alcohol is metabolized by the liver enzymes alcohol dehydrogenase and aldehyde dehydrogenase. The menstrual cycle may affect the metabolism of alcohol in women. A woman may metabolize alcohol faster during mid-cycle and may be more vulnerable to the effects of alcohol before her menstrual cycle (10).

Why the Elderly Should Drink Less

With advancing age, the activities of enzymes responsible for the metabolism of alcohol are reduced. As a result, elimination of alcohol from the body is relatively slower compared to a young individual. Lean body mass decreases and adipose (fat) tissue increases with advancing age resulting in a corresponding decrease in the volume of total body water. Therefore, an older person may experience a higher blood alcohol level than a younger person with the same body weight after drinking the same amount of alcohol because less amount of water is available in the body to dissolve alcohol (11). However, the moderate consumption of alcohol is still acceptable in elderly people unless otherwise advised by the physician. Elderly people may be taking certain medications that may interact with alcohol or they may have health issues such as liver disease that may impair alcohol metabolism.

Why Pregnant Women Should Not Drink

Pregnant women and women planning to get pregnant should not drink at all because alcohol is a known teratogen (an agent that crosses the placenta and harms the fetus). Drinking during pregnancy may cause various birth defects which are collectively called "fetal alcohol spectrum of disorders," while more serious birth defects are collectively known as "fetal alcohol syndrome." The risk of miscarriage and stillbirth are also increased significantly if a pregnant woman drinks any amount of alcohol. Drinking during pregnancy adversely affects the brain of the fetus which eventually may cause mental retardation in the child, along with behavioral and social problems. In addition, growth retardation and endocrine problems are also observed in children where the mother consumed alcohol during pregnancy. There is no safe amount of alcohol to consume during pregnancy. Therefore, a pregnant woman or a woman planning to get pregnant should not drink at all. Moreover, there is no treatment for fetal alcohol syndrome (12).

Although the harmful effect of alcohol during pregnancy is well-established, whether drinking in moderation during breastfeeding is harmful to the newborn baby or not, is not well understood. In some cultures, drinking during breastfeeding is encouraged so that a mother may produce more breast milk. However, scientific research indicates that drinking inhibits the milk ejection reflex causing a temporary decrease in milk yield. Moreover, a small amount of alcohol is present in breast milk and newborns eliminate alcohol almost at a rate of half to the adult. Minute behavioral change in infants exposed to alcohol containing milk has been reported (13). Moreover, an infant may drink less breast milk due to the alcoholic odor. Although there is no scientific consensus whether a mother should consume alcohol or not during breastfeeding, it is recommended that women should not drink during breastfeeding. When the breastfeeding period is over, a mother can resume drinking, following the guidelines for moderate alcohol consumption.

Alcohol-Medication Interactions

Certain medications (both prescription and over the counter) interact with alcohol and drinking must be avoided while taking such medications. Alcohol may alter the absorption or elimination of certain drugs (pharmacokinetic interactions) or alcohol may act in synergy with a medication (pharmacodynamic interaction). Alcohol even interacts with aspirin and with acetaminophen (the active ingredient of Tylenol) but more serious interactions occur with certain antibiotics. If a medication warning label indicates that alcohol should not be consumed when taking such medication, it is crucial to respect that warning. Many antibiotics interact with alcohol and if your doctor prescribes such antibiotics, refrain from drinking. Moreover, people taking certain medication for anxiety (alprazolam, lorazepam, temazepam, diazepam, etc.), should also avoid alcohol if recommended by their physician because in certain dosages these medications interact with alcohol, making the person drowsy which may impair their driving skills. If stopped by the police and alcohol is below the 0.08% level but such medications are present in the blood, the person may be prosecuted for Driving with Impairment (DWI).

Similar impairment may occur if a person is taking narcotic analgesics (codeine, morphine, hydrocodone, hydromorphone, oxycodone, oxymorphone, tramadol, etc.) and consumes alcohol. Therefore, commonly prescribed narcotic analgesics such as Tylenol II (acetaminophen/codeine), Vicodin (acetaminophen/hydrocodone), Dilaudid (hydromorphone), and OxyContin (oxycodone) interact with alcohol, causing increased sedation, drowsiness, and impaired motor skills. Consuming too much alcohol along with abusing these prescription medications may even cause death. Therefore, it is better to avoid alcohol when taking such medications. Common interactions between alcohol and medication are summarized in table 3.

Table 3. Common medication-alcohol interactions

Medication class	Specific examples	Comments
Antibiotics	Erythromycin, metronidazole, sulfonamides, nitrofurantoin, ornidazole, etc. (if your antibiotic medication label warns against drinking, respect that warning)	Adverse reactions if alcohol is consumed. Avoid drinking while taking such medications.
Antihistamine	Antihistamines such as diphenhydramine (Benadryl), chlorpheniramine, and hydroxyzine that cause drowsiness	Increased drowsiness and impaired driving skill if alcohol is consumed.
Nonsteroidal anti-inflammatory medications (NSAIDs)	Aspirin, ibuprofen, fenoprofen, naproxen, indomethacin, etc.	If NSAIDs are consumed for a few weeks or more, alcohol may increase the risk of gastrointestinal bleeding. However, if aspirin or ibuprofen is taken for a day of two for headache, usually there is no effect.
Benzodiazepines	Alprazolam, lorazepam, temazepam, diazepam, etc.	If alcohol is consumed while taking these medications, they may increase sedation, drowsiness, and may cause impaired driving skills.
Narcotic	Codeine, morphine,	May increase

analgesic	oxycodone, oxymorphone, hydrocodone, hydromorphone, tramadol, propoxyphene, etc.	sedation, drowsiness, and impairment of driving skills if alcohol is also consumed. Consuming too much alcohol while abusing prescription narcotic analgesics may even be fatal.
Blood pressure medication	Felodipine	Avoid consuming alcohol because that may cause lightheadedness due to a further reduction of blood pressure.

How to Estimate Blood Alcohol from the Number of Drinks, Body Weight, and Gender

Because a standard alcoholic drink contains 14 gm of alcohol, it is possible to calculate the blood alcohol level based on the number of drinks consumed, the time frame of drinking, body weight of the person and, gender. The most commonly used formula is known as the "Widmark formula" developed by the Swedish scientist, Eric P. Widmark, in 1932. The formula is as follows:

$A = C \times W \times r$

A: total amount of alcohol consumed in gm

C: blood alcohol level in gm/liter

W: body weight in kilogram and "r" is constant which is 0.7 for men and 0.6 for women.

Therefore:

$C = (A/ W \times r) - 0.015$ t, where t represents the time passed since the beginning of drinking and 0.015 factor represents the average rate of elimination of alcohol (0.015%/ per hour).

In the United States, this formula is further modified into:

C = (Number of drinks x 3.1/Weight in pounds x r) – 0.015 t (r is 0.7 for men, 0.6 for women)

Therefore, if a man with a body weight of 150 pounds consumes 3 drinks in one hour, the projected blood alcohol level, C, should be:

$C = (3 \times 3.1/150 \times 0.7) -0.015 \times 1 = 0.074$ % (legal limit of drinking 0.08%)

For a woman weighing 150 pounds and consuming 3 drinks in one hour, the projected blood alcohol level C should be:

$C = (5 \times 3.1/150 \times 0.6) -0.015 \times 0.015 = 0.088$ %

Therefore, consuming the same amount of alcohol, a woman should have higher blood alcohol than a man.

Guidelines for Safe Drinking and Avoiding DWI

In order to avoid DWI, alcohol must be sipped and be consumed with food. The projected blood alcohol after consuming 1, 2, or 3 drinks in one hour for men and women based on body weight, are listed in table 4. The blood alcohol was calculated using the Widmark formula. The overall guidelines that are recommended by this author are as follows:

•Both males and females weighing at least 100 pounds but less than 125 pounds may consume 1standard drink with food in one hour.

•Males with a body weight of 125 pounds or more may

consume 2 standard drinks with food in one hour.

•Females with a body weight of more than 125 pounds should also consume 1 standard drink with food in one hour.

Theoretically, men weighing at least 175 pounds may consume up to 3drinks in one hour and women weighing at least 200 pounds may consume up to 3 drinks in one hour and the calculated blood alcohol should be still below the legal limit of 0.08%. Moreover, any man weighing 225 pounds may consume 4drinks in one hour and the projected blood alcohol should be below the legal limit of driving. However, this practice is not safe because it violates the guidelines of the moderate consumption of alcohol. The National Institute of Alcohol Abuse and Alcoholism (NIAA) recommends that it is best not to consume any alcohol if you plan to drive. This is due to the fact that scientific research has shown that alcohol-induced impairment may start at a much lower blood alcohol level than the legal limit of driving in the United States.

Falleti et al. (2003) demonstrated that cognitive impairment associated with 0.05% blood alcohol is similar to staying awake for 24 hours (14). Moreover, many industrialized countries such as Austria, France, Germany, and Italy have set the legal limit of driving at 0.05%. Although the legal limit of driving in Canada is 0.08%, in some Canadian provinces, 0.05% blood alcohol is considered as a "warn range" limit at which an officer may suspend the driver's license for one to seven days. The National Transportation Safety Board (NTSB) in 2014, recommended lowering the legal limit of driving in the United States to 0.05% but it is not adopted as the law. Scientific research has shown that even at 0.05% blood alcohol virtually all drivers are impaired regarding at least some driving practices (15).

Table 4. Calculated blood alcohol level (expressed in nearest 2 decimal places) in men and women with various body weights after consuming 1 2, or 3 drinks in one hour (Legal Limit of Driving: 0.08%)

Body weight	Gender	Blood alcohol after 1 drink	Blood alcohol after 2 drinks	Blood alcohol after 3 drinks
100 lb	Male	0.029%	0.074%	0.117%
100 lb	Female	0.037%	0.88 %	0.14%
125 lb	Male	0.020%	0.056%	0.091%
125 lb	Female	0.026%	0.068%	0.109%
150 lb	Male	0.015%	0.044%	0.074%
150 lb	Female	0.019%	0.054%	0.088%
175 lb	Male	0.010%	0.036%	0.061%
175 lb	Female	0.014%	0.044%	0.074%
200 lb	Male	0.007%	0.029%	0.051%
200 lb	Female	0.011%	0.037%	0.063%
225 lb	Male	0.005%	0.024%	0.044%
225 lb	Female	0.008%	0.031%	0.054%
250 lb	Male	0.003%	0.025%	0.038%
250 lb	Female	0.006%	0.026%	0.047%

Note: Although these are projected blood alcohol levels based on body weight and gender, if alcohol is consumed in a 1-hour period, there are many other factors including genetic factors that may affect blood alcohol concentration.

Binge drinking (drinking at least 4 drinks in a session for females, or 5 drinks for males) is dangerous because it will always push the blood alcohol level over the legal limit of driving. In table 5, projected blood alcohol as a result of binge drinking is provided (assuming all drinks are consumed in one hour) using the Widmark formula.

Table 5. Effect of binge drinking on projected blood alcohol levels (assuming all drinks are consumed in one hour)

Body weight	Gender	Projected blood alcohol (whole blood)
100 lb	Male	0.21 %
100 lb	Female	0.24%
125 lb	Male	0.16%
125 lb	Female	0.19%
150 lb	Male	0.13%
150 lb	Female	0.16%
175 lb	Male	0.11%
175 lb	Female	0.13%
200 lb	Male	0.096%
200 lb	Female	0.11%
225 lb	Male	0.083%
225 lb	Female	0.10%
250 lb	Male	0.074%
250 lb	Female	0.088%

Breathalyzers versus Blood Alcohol Determination

Breathalyzers estimate blood alcohol content from the concentration of alcohol in the breath. The estimated ratio between breath alcohol and blood alcohol is 1:2100. Therefore, multiplying breath alcohol concentration by 2100 provides blood alcohol in mg/L (or multiplying by 210 to get blood alcohol in mg/dL). In general, Breathalyzer software automatically calculates blood alcohol values from observed breath alcohol levels. Breathalyzers are based on various technologies:

- Colorimetric method based on the chemical reaction of alcohol with a cocktail of chemicals
- Infrared spectroscopy technology
- Fuel cell technology
- Mixed technology (fuel cell and infrared).

Breathalyzers may be evidentiary Breathalyzers (approved by the National Highway Traffic Safety Administration) which are usually used by police officers to determine the blood alcohol level of a suspected impaired driver. The results of an evidentiary Breathalyzer are accepted as evidence by the court of law; the blood alcohol level may not be needed for prosecution. There are also non-evidentiary Breathalyzers. Personal Breathalyzers, which are commercially available, are not evidentiary Breathalyzers but may be cleared by the FDA for sale to the public.

There are several different brands of evidentiary breath alcohol analyzers which are based on the principle of fuel cell technology, for example, Alcotest Models 6510, 6810, and 7410 (National Drager, Durango, Colorado), and Alco-Sensor III and IV (Intoximeters Inc., St. Louis, MO) while other evidentiary breath analyzers are based on mixed technology (both fuel cell and infrared spectroscopy). Fuel cell technology is considered superior to other technologies for Breathalyzers. Personal Breathalyzers, for example, various BACTrack brands of Breathalyzers are based on fuel cell technology.

. When performing a breath alcohol test, the subject is asked to inhale ambient air and to exhale into the breath analyzer (usually 1.1 to 1.5 L of exhaled air is needed for the test). Therefore, a smaller subject with a smaller lung capacity must exhale a greater fraction of air in their lungs to fulfill the minimum volume requirement of the analyzer and as a result, the alcohol breath test may overestimate the blood alcohol level in smaller subjects compared to larger subjects with larger lung capacities (16).

There are other issues with Breathalyzers that may produce misleading readings. Sometimes a driver stopped by the police may use a mouthwash to hide any alcoholic breath. Because some mouthwashes contain alcohol, the use of a mouthwash prior to taking a breath alcohol test may cause falsely elevated breath alcohol results. However, residual alcohol evaporates from the mouth rapidly and a mandatory 15-minute waiting time in the police station when no food or drink is allowed, eliminates the possibility of a false result. Some energy drinks contain low amounts of alcohol, but again, a 15-minute waiting time is sufficient to eliminate the possibility of a false positive test result using a Breathalyzer. Breathalyzers cannot differentiate between the use of methanol (wood alcohol) and ethyl alcohol (alcohol). However, methanol abuse is dangerous as it may cause blindness. In addition, consuming the ketogenic diet may cause false positive test results. Glue sniffing may also cause false positive breath alcohol. Common interferences in breath alcohol analyzers are summarized in table 6.

Table 6. Falsely elevated results using Breathalyzers

•In some individuals breath alcohol may peak 30-40 minutes after their last drink. Therefore, the best practice is to finish your alcohol drink and then eat the rest of your food.

•Methanol poisoning may be mistakenly identified as blood alcohol using Breathalyzers. However, drinking methanol instead of alcohol is dangerous because methanol may cause blindness.

•Ketogenic diets may produce false positive alcohol results using Breathalyzers.

•Glue sniffing is a dangerous practice and it may produce false positive Breathalyzer results.

Blood alcohol may be measured in serum (the aqueous layer of the blood which is separated from blood cells) or in whole blood. In crime and forensic toxicology laboratories, whole blood alcohol is measured using headspace-gas chromatography which is the gold standard of blood alcohol measurement. In hospital laboratories alcohol is measured in the serum using enzymatic methods and automated chemistry analyzers. Serum alcohol is always higher than whole blood alcohol because of its higher water content. This alcohol must be multiplied by 0.87 in order to get whole blood alcohol because the legal limit of driving is

0.08% whole blood alcohol. For example, if serum alcohol is 90 mg/dL (0.09%), then whole blood alcohol is 78 mg/dL (0.078%).

If stopped by the police for suspected driving under the influence of alcohol, always insist for a blood alcohol analysis because blood alcohol is always accurate if performed by headspace gas chromatography in a forensic or crime laboratory. First, this will give you some time because some alcohol should be metabolized between being stopped by the police and blood drawn in a police station or in another facility. For example, if someone has a blood alcohol level of 0.09% when stopped by the police and blood is drawn an hour later, the blood alcohol should be reduced to 0.075% (blood alcohol is reduced by 0.015% per hour). If the person is prosecuted, a discrepancy between Breathalyzer value and blood alcohol value, which is below the legal limit, may give the defense attorney a chance to raise doubts about the true blood alcohol in the minds of jury members. For conviction in a DWI case, the burden of proof without any reasonable doubt is on the prosecution.

The guidelines provided in this chapter are very conservative to avoid DWI. If you drink more than what is recommended based on your body weight and gender, the recommendation is to use a personal Breathalyzer before you drive. There are many limitations of personal Breathalyzers but if the personal Breathalyzer is properly calibrated or recalibrated by the manufacturer and if the breath alcohol analysis shows a value of 0.06% or less, then it may be safe to drive. If the value is close to 0.075%, it is advisable to wait for 30-40 minutes. Also, breath alcohol may peak 30-40 minutes after the last drink in some individuals. It will be best to finish the drink before finishing your meal and take some time before driving to be on the safe side.

Mixing Illicit Drugs with Alcohol: A Deadly Combination

Alcohol interacts with narcotic pain analgesics and benzodiazepines. Therefore, alcohol should be avoided if you are taking such medications. However, consuming heavy amounts of alcohol with narcotic pain medications (opioids) or benzodiazepines, may precipitate a severe drug overdose. Abusing alcohol and narcotic pain medication may also cause fatalities. Mixing illicit drugs such as cocaine with alcohol is a deadly combination due to the formation of cocaethylene, a very toxic metabolite of cocaine. Alcohol lowers the threshold of fatal toxic levels of many illicit drugs including cocaine, amphetamines, barbiturates, benzodiazepines, opioids, phencyclidine, and various designer drugs (including bath salts and spices) that are abused.

Conclusions

Drinking alcohol in moderation has many health benefits, but all such benefits disappear when a person drinks in excess. Consuming alcohol in moderation also helps a person to relax and to socialize because alcohol may reduce their inhibition. Even consuming half of the drink is enough to get the pleasurable effects because even at a very low blood level, the pleasurable effects of alcohol can be experienced. Drinking alcohol in a social context (social drinkers) even once a week where just 1 standard drink is consumed, is good for health. However, the pleasurable effects of alcohol disappear with increasing blood alcohol levels and at higher doses alcohol acts as a poison.

3 HEALTH BENEFITS OF DRINKING IN MODERATION

Introduction

Social drinkers and moderate drinkers are blessed with the many health benefits of alcohol. The guidelines for moderate drinking recommend the consumption of up to 2 alcoholic beverages a day for a man but up to 1 alcoholic beverage a day for a woman. Any individual drinking more than these guidelines is considered heavy drinking. This can be understood simply by considering alcohol as a legal over-the-counter medication. By definition, a medication if taken in the recommended dosage provides benefits, but if taken in more than the recommended dosage is a poison. In one study the authors showed that even consuming large but tolerable amounts of alcohol in one session may trigger the onset of embolic stroke (when a blood clot is formed elsewhere in the body but travels to the brain causing stroke) and acute myocardial infarction (heart attack) (1). Interestingly, when alcohol is consumed in moderation, it protects the heart and reduces the probability of a heart attack. The guidelines for consuming alcohol in moderation are given in table 1.

Table 1. Guidelines for moderate consumption of alcohol

•Men: Up to 2 drinks a day

•Women: Up to 1 drink a day

One drink is defined as containing 14 gm (0.6 fl oz) of alcohol. The one alcoholic drink is equivalent to drinking 12 fl oz of regular beer (5% alcohol), 5 fl oz of wine (12% alcohol), or 1.5 fl oz of 80 proof-distilled spirits (40% alcohol).

The FDA does not consider mixing alcohol and caffeine as a safe practice. People who mix alcohol and caffeine may drink more alcohol and become more intoxicated than they realize, increasing the risk of alcohol-related adverse events.

The benefits of consuming alcohol in moderation are both physical and mental. The best benefit is the protection of the heart thus reducing the incidence of cardiovascular diseases. However, moderate alcohol consumption also reduces the risk of stroke. The major mental health benefit of alcohol if consumed in moderation, is that it is very effective in reducing stress. In older people, moderate drinking also has protective effects against developing depression. Interestingly, older men (50 years of age or older) get more benefits from consuming alcohol in moderation compared to younger men. However, women of any age get health benefits from consuming moderate amounts of alcohol. Some benefits of drinking in moderation are attributable to alcohol while other benefits are due to the combined effect of both alcohol and many beneficial organic compounds present in beer and in wine. More than 400 different phytochemicals are present in beer; some of these compounds originate from raw materials while others are generated during the fermentation process. Melatonin is generated during the brewing process (2). More than 1,600 phytochemicals are present in wine prepared from grapes (3).

Moderate Alcohol Consumption Protects the Heart

Probably the number one benefit of drinking in

moderation is the reduced risk of developing cardiovascular diseases including heart attacks. However, heavy drinking is associated with heart diseases because alcohol in higher concentrations damages the heart. The first report that moderate alcohol consumption protects the heart came from the Framingham Heart Study. This study was initiated in 1948, where investigators recruited 5,209 men and women between the ages of 30 and 62 from the town of Framingham, Massachusetts. The Framingham Heart Study was conducted under the direction of the National Heart, Lung and Blood Institute (an institute affiliated with the National Institute of Health). The study is also active today and results of these studies identified many risk factors for heart diseases and for other diseases. Many guidelines published by the American Heart Association and by other professional societies are results of observations published by researchers of the Framingham Heart Study in prestigious medical journals.

The relationship between alcohol consumption and cardiovascular diseases was examined in the original Framingham Heart Study which showed a U shape curve indicating that moderate alcohol consumption was associated with a reduced risk of developing cardiovascular diseases but heavy alcohol consumption increased this risk. Smoking is a risk factor for developing cardiovascular diseases but moderate alcohol consumption may also provide some protection even in smokers (4). Interestingly, women just need to drink once a week for protection from heart diseases while men may need to drink 1 standard drink every day to get the same benefits. These findings were based on a study where the authors enrolled 28,448 women and 25,052 men between 50 and 65 years of age who were free from cardiovascular diseases at the time of enrollment, and then conducted a follow-up for 5.7 years. The authors observed little differences between women who consumed at least 1 drink per week compared to women who consumed 2-4 drinks per week, 5-6 drinks per week, or even

7 drinks per week. For men, the lowest risk was found in individuals who consumed 1drink per day (5).

O'Keefe et al. (2014) reviewed the effect of alcohol on the health of the human heart and commented that habitual light to moderate drinking lowers the rate from death due to coronary artery disease (heart attacks are coronary artery diseases where plaque formation in the arteries and eventually a blood clot significantly reduces or prevents the blood going to the heart); diabetes mellitus (the most common form of diabetes which is either due to insulin resistance or reduced/impaired production of insulin by the pancreas); congestive heart failure; and stroke. However, excessive alcohol consumption is the third leading cause of premature death in the United States. In general, men older than age 50 gets more favorable effects of consuming alcohol in moderation than younger men but women of any age get favorable effects. Unfortunately, cardioprotective effects of alcohol has not been documented in epidemiological studies of populations from India and from China. The authors advise people to drink 1 glass of red wine (5- 6- oz glass) daily immediately before or during dinner. However, the authors also advise individuals who are teetotalers not to initiate light to moderate alcohol consumption for health benefits because of the paucity of randomized outcome data and the potential for developing problem drinking practices (6). Gemes et al. (2016), based on a study of 58,827 individuals and 11.6 year follow-ups, observed that light to moderate consumption of alcohol was associated with a lower risk of heart attacks (7).

Light to moderate consumption of alcohol also increases the chance of survival after the first heart attack. Based on a study of 1,253 women who survived their first acute heart attacks, Rosenbloom et al. (2012) observed that compared to women who did not drink at all, women who consumed less than 1 drink per week, 1to 3 drinks per week, or more than 3drinks per week, all showed lower mortality in a 10-year follow-up. All types of alcoholic beverages (beer, wine, or liquor) were associated with the protection. The authors estimated that light to moderate consumption of alcohol by women after their first heart attacks was associated with approximately a 35% lower chance of dying compared to women who did not consume any alcohol (8).

In general, light to moderate consumption of beer or wine is better than drinking rum, vodka, or whiskey to get protection from cardiovascular diseases although drinking any alcoholic beverage in moderation protects the heart. However, an important phenomenon known as the "French paradox" (there is a low incidence of cardiovascular diseases in the French population despite eating fatty food) is related to the regular consumption of red wine by French people. The superiority of red wine in reducing risks of cardiovascular diseases compared to other alcoholic beverages may be attributable to grape-derived natural products such as resveratrol which is present in red wine in significant amounts (9).

There are several hypotheses on how moderate drinking can reduce the risk of developing cardiovascular diseases. In general, at moderate concentrations, alcohol increases the concentration of good cholesterol known as HDL-cholesterol (high-density lipoprotein cholesterol) in the blood. Because this increase is totally attributable to alcohol, consuming any alcoholic beverages in moderation is associated with good cardiac health. However, studies have also indicated that the level of increase in HDL cholesterol in the blood may explain 50% of the protective effect of alcohol against cardiovascular diseases and the other 50% may be partly related to antioxidant, anti-inflammatory, and anti-platelet effects (anti-platelet effects reduces the risk of blood clot formation) of beneficial compounds other than alcohol which are present in beer and wine but not in distilled liquors such as vodka, rum, or whiskey. These beneficial organic compounds are known as polyphenolic and phenolic compounds. These chemicals are naturally present in barley, hops, and grapes. However, for preparing distilled liquor, for example, whiskey, which can be made from barley, corn, rye, or wheat, polyphenolic compounds are present in the original grain from which whiskey is initially fermented but during the distillation process, these chemicals are lost. However, during the aging of distilled liquors using wood barrels, some polyphenolic compounds present in the wood may leak into the distilled liquor.

Moderate Alcohol Consumption Reduces the Risk of Stroke

Another beneficial effect of consuming alcohol in moderation is the reduction in the risk of stroke in both men and women regardless of age or ethnicity. The Copenhagen City Heart Study with 13,329 eligible men and women aged between 45 to 84 years with 16 years of follow-ups, demonstrated that individuals who consumed low to moderate amounts of alcohol had a lower risk of stroke but heavy alcohol consumption increased the risk of stroke (10).

Based on a study of 3,176 elderly men and women (mean age: 69.1 years), Elkind et al. (2006) observed that moderate drinkers (2 or less drinks per day; beer, wine, or liquor) had approximately a 50% less risk of having ischemic stroke (approximately 85% of strokes are ischemic stroke where the artery that supplies oxygen rich blood to the brain is blocked) compared to nondrinkers. The maximum protection was observed in individuals who consumed only 1.2 drinks per day. The authors also observed that moderate alcohol consumption protects an individual from heart attacks and from death from vascular diseases (vascular diseases are diseases of the blood vessels: arteries and veins which form the blood circulation system in the body; cardiovascular diseases including heart attacks are a subset of vascular diseases). The protective effects of moderate alcohol consumption from ischemic stroke was clearly observed in individuals who consumed alcohol in the past year but whether former drinkers who did not consume alcohol during the study also received the protective effect of alcohol or not was not clear. However, consuming more than 2 drinks a day was associated with a trend toward an increased risk of hemorrhagic stroke (less common but occurs when an artery in the brain leaks blood or ruptures) (11).

In another study, the authors also observed that the upper limit of consumption of alcohol for reducing the risk of ischemic stroke was 2 drinks a day. The protective effect of alcohol was observed in both younger and older groups; in men and women; and in Whites, Blacks, and Hispanics. Although some studies have suggested that wine may have more effects than beer or liquors, the authors in this study observed that wine, beer, and liquor had approximately the same effects although wine drinkers on average, consumed less alcohol. However, no study among Japanese subjects has shown protective effects of alcohol in ischemic stroke (12).

Moderate Alcohol Consumption Reduces the Risk of Type 2 Diabetes

There are two types of diabetes; diabetes mellitus and diabetes insipidus. Diabetes insipidus is a relatively rare disease (3 cases per 100,000 people) with a childhood onset and characterized by excessive thirst and production of diluted urine. The most common form of diabetes insipidus is the central or neurologic form which is due to a deficiency of the antidiuretic hormone (also known as "arginine vasopressin") which is secreted by the pituitary gland located in the brain. The less common form known as "nephrogenic diabetes" insipidus is due to the insensitivity of kidneys to antidiuretic hormone. Diabetes mellitus is more common and can be either Type 1(childhood onset where the pancreas produces little or no insulin) or Type 2 (adult onset where muscles cannot process insulin properly or insulin production by the pancreas is not sufficient). Moderate alcohol consumption reduces the risk of developing Type 2 diabetes but has no effect on Type 1 diabetes.

The moderate consumption of alcohol reduces the risk of developing Type 2 diabetes most probably by reducing oxidative stress and by increasing insulin sensitivity. Based on 15 studies conducted in the United States, Finland, Netherland, Germany, the United Kingdom, and Japan with 369,862 men and women and an average follow-up of 12 years, light and moderate drinkers had approximately a 30% lower risk of developing Type 2 diabetes compared to non-drinkers. It made little difference whether an individual consumed beer, wine, or spirit. However, the authors recommended consuming alcohol frequently (e.g., daily or several times in one week) rather than occasionally (13).

Light to moderate drinking (5-30 gm, 1/2 a drink to 2 drinks a day) reduces the risk of Type 2 diabetes by approximately 30%. However, drinking 48 gm or more alcohol per day (3.5 drinks or more) significantly increases the risk of Type 2 diabetes. Occasional binge drinking is also associated with an increased risk. When healthy subjects consumed wine, beer, or gin as pre-meal drinks and during the meal, postprandial blood glucose (glucose level after consuming a meal) was 16-37% lower compared to consuming similar meals with the same calories without alcohol. This indicates that alcohol may increase insulin secretion thus lowering blood glucose. Alcohol may also improve insulin sensitivity so that muscles can burn glucose more effectively for energy. However, alcohol consumption may cause low glucose levels in individuals who have Type 2 diabetes but who are also taking sulfonylurea medications (e.g., glipizide, glyburide, glimepiride, or tolbutamide) to lower blood glucose (14).

Moderate Alcohol Consumption Reduces the Risk of Certain Types of Cancer

The moderate consumption of alcohol may reduce the risk of certain types of cancer because wine and beer contain anti carcinogenic (anticancer) compounds and antioxidants.

Oxidative stress is one of the causes of cancer. Therefore, antioxidants have protective effects. In the California Men's Health Study using 84,170 men aged between 45 and 69, consumption of 1or more drinks of red wine per day was associated with approximately 60% reduced lung cancer risk in smokers (15). Consumption of up to 1drink per day reduced the risk of head and neck cancer in both men and women but consuming more than 3 alcoholic beverages increased the risk of developing cancer. In an Italian study the authors observed that moderate consumption of alcohol reduced the risk of developing renal cell carcinoma in both males and females (16).

There is a consensus that heavy alcohol consumption significantly increases the risk of breast cancer. In general, having 1 additional drink per day increases the risk from 2to 12%. However, the relation between moderate alcohol consumption and the risk of breast cancer is controversial because there are conflicting reports in the medical literature. Pelucchi et al. (2008) concluded that consumption of fewer than 3 alcoholic drinks per week is not associated with an increased risk of breast cancer, but consuming 3 to 6drinks per week may be associated with a small increase in risk (17). Lowry et al. (2016), based on a study of 7,835 women who had breast cancer, concluded that consumption of alcohol before and after breast cancer diagnosis did not increase the risk of overall or cause specific mortality (18). Interestingly, alcohol is not associated with an increased risk of all types of breast cancer. Strumylaite et al. (2015) observed that moderate alcohol consumption (up to 5 drinks per week to more than 5 drinks per week) is associated with the risk of estrogen receptor positive breast cancer, particularly in postmenopausal women (19). Beverage type is not associated with an increased risk of breast cancer because alcohol acts as a weak breast carcinogen. Moreover, alcohol may increase the responsiveness of estrogen receptors present in the breast. Acetaldehyde, a metabolite of alcohol is also a carcinogen. However, there are many other factors that may increase the risk of breast cancer including family history (BRCA1 and BRCA2 gene mutation are most common inherited factors), being older (only 10-15% breast cancer diagnoses are among women 45 years or younger), using hormone replacement therapy, used or using birth control pills, not having a child, or having a dense breast.

Other Physical Health Benefits

Moderate alcohol consumption reduces the risk of developing rheumatoid arthritis. Results from two Scandinavian studies indicated that among moderate drinkers, the risk of rheumatoid arthritis was significantly reduced. (20). Nissen et al. (2010) reported, based on a study using 2,908 patients suffering from rheumatoid arthritis, that occasional or daily consumption of alcohol reduced the progression of the disease based on radiological studies (x-ray). The best results were observed in male patients (21). In another study involving 34,141 women, the risk of rheumatoid arthritis was reduced by 37% in women who consumed more than 4 drinks per week compared to women who consumed less than 1drink per week as well as nondrinkers. Drinking all types of alcohol (beer, wine, and liquor) was associated with a reduced risk of rheumatoid arthritis (22).

Moderate drinking (5-7 drinks per week) but not light drinking (1-2 drinks per week) may reduce the risk of gallstone disease. All alcoholic beverages types are associated with a decreased risk (23). The relation between moderate alcohol consumption and the reduced risk of the common cold has been studied. In a large study using 4,272 faculty and staff of five Spanish universities as subjects, the investigators observed that total alcohol intake from drinking beer and spirits had no protective effect against the common cold whereas moderate wine consumption was associated with a reduced risk (24).

Because a moderate consumption of alcohol can prevent

many diseases, it is expected that moderate drinkers may live longer than lifetime abstainers of alcohol. Klatsky et al. (1981) studied a 10- year mortality in relation to alcohol in 8,060 subjects and observed that persons who consumed 2drinks or less daily fared best and had significant reductions in mortality rates than nondrinkers. The heaviest drinkers (6 or more drinks a day) had much higher mortality rates than moderate drinkers, while people who drink 3 to 5 drinks per day had a similar mortality rate as nondrinkers. Therefore, consuming 2 or less drinks per day is the best practice (25).

In the Physician's Health Study involving 22,071 male physicians in the United States between ages 40 and 84 with no history of myocardial infarction, stroke, or cancer, and then 10 years of follow-ups, the authors observed that men who consumed 2 to 6 drinks per week had the most favorable results (20-28% lower mortality rate) than people who consumed 1drink per week. In contrast, people who consumed more than 2 drinks per day had approximately a 50% chance of higher mortality than people who consumed just 1 drink per week (26). However, some studies indicate that wine drinkers have lower mortality than people who drink beer or spirit (see chapter 6). The physical health benefits of drinking in moderation are summarized in table 2.

Table 2. Physical health benefits of consuming alcohol in moderation

Health benefit	Type of alcoholic beverage and quantity	Comments
Reduced risk of cardiovascular diseases including heart attacks and heart failure	Beer and wine provides better protection than liquors. One author suggested drinking 1glass of red wine before or with the evening meal.	Alcohol in moderate concentration increases good cholesterol but phenolic and polyphenolic compounds present in beer and in wine

	Women may get the protection from drinking as little as 1drink per week.	may also provide additional protection. Protection is more significant in men 50 years of age and older but women of any age may get benefits of consuming alcohol in moderation.
Reduces mortality in survivors of heart attacks	Women who consume any alcoholic beverage (beer, wine, or liquor) in moderation (1 drink per week, 1-3 drinks per week, or more than 3 drinks per week) live longer after surviving their first heart attack compared to nondrinkers.	Alcohol is responsible for the protection.
Reduced risk of ischemic stroke	In one study, the authors observed maximum protection from the daily consumption of 1.2 standard drinks. Any alcoholic beverage (beer, wine, or liquor) can provide the protection if consumed in moderation.	Drinking more than 2 standard drinks a day may increase the risk of hemorrhagic stroke.
Reduced risk of Type 2 diabetes	Any alcoholic beverage (beer, wine, or liquor) can provide the protection if consumed in moderation (1/2 a	Alcohol reduces blood glucose (sugar) after a meal by stimulating insulin secretion but also may improve insulin

	drink to up to 2 drinks a day).	sensitivity. However, for individuals taking sulfonylurea medication, alcohol may cause low blood sugar (hypoglycemia).
Protection from certain types of cancer	Red wine (1 drink a day) may reduce the risk of lung cancer even in smokers. One drink a day reduces the risk of head and neck cancer as well as renal cell carcinoma.	Antioxidants present in alcoholic drinks may provide the protection but alcohol itself is a weak breast carcinogen. Even moderate drinking may increase the risk of estrogen positive breast cancer but fewer than 3 drinks per week may not be associated with an increased risk.
Reduced risk of developing rheumatoid arthritis	Moderate consumption of any type of alcoholic beverage reduces the risk of rheumatoid arthritis.	Alcohol may reduce the generation of molecules that cause inflammation.
Reduced risk of forming gallstones	Consuming 5-7 drinks (any type of alcoholic beverage) per week reduces the risk of gallstone disease.	People who are light drinkers (consuming 1-2 drinks per week) may not get any protection from gallstone disease.
Protection from the common cold	Beer and sprit have no protective effect but moderate wine consumption may protect from the common cold.	Probably some specific polyphenolic compounds present in wine provides the protection.
Increased	One or 2drinks a day	Overall effect of

longevity	may increase longevity but drinking more than 2 drinks a day may reduce longevity.	alcohol and antioxidants present in beer and wine may be responsible for a longer life in moderate drinkers. Drinking wine may have an additional benefit for longevity.

Mental Health Benefits of Moderate Drinking

Alcohol, if consumed in moderation, not only produces mild euphoria and relaxation, but also reduces stress. Moreover, alcohol can reduce the risk of developing age-related dementia and Alzheimer's disease. However, it is important not to start drinking before 21 because the onset of drinking at an early age (13 or earlier) has devastating effects on the brain and such adverse effects may last a lifetime in such individuals. Underage drinkers are also susceptible to the immediate ill effects of alcohol use such as blackouts, hangovers, and alcohol poisoning and these individuals are also at a higher risk of neurodegeneration, impairment of functional brain activity, and neurocognitive deficits. Women are more susceptible to alcohol-related neurological damage than men, because a female adolescent brain is more vulnerable to alcohol exposure that a male adolescent brain (see chapter 4 for more details).

People like to drink alcohol because of its ability to modify emotional states. Alcohol has a euphoric effect at a low to moderate blood alcohol (0.02 to 0.05% whole blood alcohol levels) concentrations and such effect starts 10-15 minutes after the initiation of drinking. Alcohol is known to cause a reduction in inhibition and that loss of inhibition after drinking is most significant in females compared to males. In one study based on 184 degree-level and postgraduate students (94 females, 90 males) indicated that alcohol at a level of approximately 50 mg/dL (0.05%)

facilitated social interaction and communication (27).

Moderate alcohol consumption is very effective in reducing stress and self-perception of good health. In general, consuming 3 to 9 drinks per week is associated with a self-perception of good health and wellbeing. Subjective health may simply be an indicator of actual health status and moderate consumption of alcohol may provide a rewarding sense of wellbeing in association with good physical health. Moderate drinking is also associated with stress reduction, mood enhancement, sociability, social integration, and improvement in cognitive function. A possible link between moderate drinking and success at work may be related to overall better physical health, better psychosocial adjustment for the individual as well as greater involvement in employment-related social experiences. Moreover, during stressful work environments, nondrinkers are more likely to be absent from work than moderate drinkers. Alcohol may have a buffering effect between stress and sickness. Moreover, nondrinkers are 27% more likely to be disabled compared to moderate drinkers. Incidentally, studies have shown that moderate drinkers may have higher incomes than teetalers (28). A Spanish study reported that moderate alcohol consumption, especially drinking wine, was associated with more active lifestyles and better perception of health in elderly subjects (29). Studies have shown that moderate alcohol consumption is associated with reduced depression in elderly subjects. However, heavy drinking is associated with higher rates of clinical depression.

Age-related dementia and Alzheimer's disease are neurodegenerative diseases associated with advanced age. Alzheimer's disease is a devastating neurological disorder affecting 1 in 10 Americans over the age of 65 and almost half of all Americans over 85 years old. Moderate alcohol consumption can dramatically reduce the risk of age-related dementia and Alzheimer's disease. The triggering agent for Alzheimer's disease is β-amyloid peptide (Aβ-aggregates) which alters the synaptic activity and disrupts neurotransmission mediated by N-methyl–D-aspartate receptor in the brain. Alcohol in low dosages can prevent the formation of Aβ-aggregates, thus delaying or preventing the onset of Alzheimer's disease. Moreover, low to moderate consumption of alcohol is also associated with a reduced risk of other neurodegenerative diseases as evidenced from data of several large clinical trials (30). Dietary compounds (polyphenols) found in grapes have some protective effect from Alzheimer's disease because these compounds interfere with generation and aggregation of β-amyloid peptide. Resveratrol, a compound found in abundance in red wine and also in grapes, provides protection from Alzheimer's disease (31). The mental health benefits of drinking in moderation are summarized in table 3.

Table 3. Mental health benefits of consuming alcohol in moderation

•Stress reduction and overall perception of good health

•Mood enhancement, sociability, and social integration

•Alcohol in low concentration (0.05% or less) reduces inhibition but mostly in women

•Some improvement in cognitive function including short-term memory

•Better performance at work and fewer sick leaves

•Reduced risk of depression especially in older people

•Reduced risk of developing age-related dementia and Alzheimer's disease (red wine may be more effective) in the elderly

Conclusions

The moderate consumption of alcohol is associated with many health benefits but one of the major benefits is protection from cardiovascular diseases including heart attacks and heart failure. Moreover, moderate consumption of alcohol is also associated with the reduced risk of stroke, Type 2 diabetes, certain type of cancer, rheumatoid arthritis, and gallstone disease. Moderate alcohol consumption may also increase longevity and red wine may provide protection from the common cold. However, the relationship between moderate alcohol consumption and cancer is controversial especially for breast cancer. Nevertheless, Pelucchi et al. (2008) concluded that drinking less than 3drinks per week is not associated with an increased risk of breast cancer. Women get health benefits of alcohol just from 1-2 drinks per week. Moderate alcohol consumption is also associated with stress release, improved mood, better social interaction, lesser days of missed work, and an overall perception of good health. Moderate drinking, especially drinking red wine, is associated with a reduced risk of age-related dementia and Alzheimer's disease.

4 HAZARDS OF DRINKING IN EXCESS

Introduction

In chapter 3, the many health benefits of drinking in moderation were discussed. Unfortunately, all of these benefits disappear with the heavy consumption of alcohol. Heavy alcohol consumption may lead to alcohol dependence which is referred to as "alcohol use disorder." This is a psychiatric illness similar to substance abuse (illicit or prescription drug abuse). Alcohol, if consumed in moderation, is like a medicine but medicines become poisons if taken in excess dosage. Therefore, treat alcohol with respect and avoid misuse.

The best effect of consuming alcohol in moderation is protection from cardiovascular diseases, but with excess consumption, alcohol acts as a toxin to the heart thus increasing the risk of cardiovascular diseases including heart failure and heart attacks. However, the most common adverse effects of alcohol are on the liver. Excess alcohol consumption is associated with liver diseases including cirrhosis of the liver. Alcohol damages the human immune system, making an individual more susceptible to infection. Alcohol abuse also damages the endocrine system and increases the risk of cancer and is associated with a reduced lifespan, depression, marital problems, domestic abuse, violent crime, and homicide. A person may also die from alcohol poisoning.

Definition of Binge Drinking and Heavy Drinking

As discussed in chapter 2, moderate drinking is consuming up to 2 standard drinks for males, up to 1 standard drink for females. Any individual consuming alcohol more than these limits can be considered as heavy drinkers.

Binge drinking is defined by the National Institute of Alcohol Abuse and Alcoholism (NIAAA) as consumption of 5 drinks in 2 hours for men, and 4 drinks in the same time period for women and such drinking process always produce a blood alcohol level of 0.08% or higher. However, another government agency, the Substance Abuse and Mental Health Services Administration (SAMHSA) defines binge drinking as consuming 5or more alcoholic beverages on the same occasion in the past 30 days during their survey regarding alcohol and drug abuse patterns. SAMHSA also defines heavy drinking as consuming 5 or more drinks on the same occasion on each of 5 or more days in the past 30 days. NIAAA investigators also showed that if women consume 3 drinks on a single day not exceeding 7 drinks a week and men consume 4 drinks on a single occasion but not exceeding 14 drinks per week, the possibility of developing alcohol use disorder (AUD) is approximately 2%, a relatively low risk for developing AUD. The definitions of moderate, binge, heavy, and underage drinking are listed in table 1.

Table 1. Definition of moderate, heavy, risky, and binge drinking

Type of drinking*	Gender	Definition/guideline
Moderate drinking	Men	Up to 2 drinks a day
Moderate drinking	Women	Up to 1 drink per day

Heavy drinking	Men	Consuming 15 or more drinks per week
Heavy drinking	Women	Consuming 8 or more drinks per week
Heavy drinking (SAMHSA) guideline	Both men and women	Consuming 5 or more drinks in the same occasion on each of 5 or more days in the past 30 days
Binge drinking	Men	Consuming 5 drinks in a 2-hour period
Binge drinking	Women	Consuming 4 drinks in a 2-hour period
Binge drinking (SAMHSA)	Both men and women	Consuming 5 or more drinks in the same occasion at least 1 day in the past 30 days
Underage drinking	Both men and women	Legal age of drinking in all states in the United States is 21 years. Anyone drinking below that age is considered as underage drinking. Many states have zero tolerance law for underage drinking and anyone below 21 years of age stopped by the police with suspected DWI may be prosecuted even if blood alcohol is well below the legal limit of 0.08%.

*USDA/NIH 2015-2000 Dietary guidelines
SAMHSA: Substance Abuse and Mental Health Services Administration

There is a misconception that if the number of total drinks in a week does not exceed 14 for men and 7 drinks for women, then the drinking practice is safe. However, consuming 4 drinks on Friday, 5 drinks on both Saturday and Sunday, but not drinking on other days of the week (total alcohol consumption per week: 14 standard drinks) by a male is not considered as a safe drinking practice. In fact, the person is binge drinking on both Saturday and Sunday. Irregular binge drinking even once a month increases the risk of cardiovascular diseases rather than protecting the heart as observed in moderate drinkers. The cardioprotective effect of moderate drinking also disappears when light to moderate drinking is mixed with occasional heavy drinking episodes (1). Another obvious complication of binge drinking is facing a charge of DWI if stopped by the police because binge drinking always results in blood alcohol over the legal limit of driving. Studies have also shown that even occasional binge drinking is associated with an increased risk of stroke, alcoholic hepatitis, pancreatitis, and heart attacks. More frequent binge drinking is associated with the risk of developing alcohol abuse, poor job performance, spouse abuse, divorce, and depression.

Despite having a legal drinking age of 21 in the United States, binge drinking is very popular among high school and college students. Miller et al. (2007) reported that overall, 44.9% of high school students surveyed, reported drinking in the past 30 days including 28.8% who were binge drinkers. Binge drinking rates increased with age and school grade. These drinkers also reported poor performance in school and involvement with risky behaviors such as riding with a driver who had been drinking, being sexually active, smoking cigarettes, using illicit drugs, attempting suicide, and being a victim of dating violence (2). Predictably, college binge drinkers are more likely than their nondrinking counterparts to experience one or more alcohol-related problems while in college. In addition, in one study the authors observed in a 10-year follow-up of binge drinkers, that such drinkers had a much higher risk of becoming dependent on alcohol later in life. Binge drinking also caused an early departure from college and less favorable labor market outcomes (3). The human brain is still developing during adolescent years and underage drinking has devastating effects on their brains.

When adults are involved in binge drinking they may

consume an average of 8 drinks. In one study, the authors found that 74.4% of adult binge drinkers consumed beer exclusively or predominately, and 80.5% of binge drinkers consumed at least some beer. Wine accounted for only 10.9% of binge drinks consumed (4). As expected, binge drinking is associated with higher mortality rates. In one study the authors observed higher all-cause mortality in males and females as well as higher mortality among men due to cardiovascular diseases in binge drinkers compared to non-binge drinkers (5). Although pregnant women should not drink at all, studies have shown that pregnant women who were involved in occasional binge drinking episodes had much higher risks of stillbirth as well as sudden deaths of infants.

Alcohol Use Disorder

Alcohol abuse and alcoholism are psychiatric illnesses requiring treatment but if treated properly (using medication and/or counseling) this illness can be cured. Before 2013, there were two illnesses; alcohol abuse and alcohol dependence dealing with the excessive consumption of alcohol. In 2013, the American Psychiatric Association issued the 5th edition of *Diagnostics and Statistical Manual of Mental Disorders* (DSM-5), where both disorders were categorized under one disorder called "Alcohol Use Disorder" or AUD. AUD can be mild, moderate, or severe based on diagnostic criteria. Anyone meeting 2of the 11 criteria in the past 12 months is considered as having AUD. If 2 to3 criteria are present AUD is mild, if 4 to 5 criteria are present, the AUD is moderate, but if 6 or more criteria are present, then AUD is considered as severe. Even if mild AUD is present, medical intervention is warranted. The diagnosis of AUD is based on the interview of the patient with a qualified physician or with a health care professional. Some signs and symptoms of AUD are listed:

•Being unable to stop drinking even when one wishes to stop

•Unable to cut the number of drinks due to an uncontrollable urge to drink (indicating alcohol dependence)

•Consuming more alcohol now than when drinking was initiated because the same number of drinks no longer produces desired effects (alcohol tolerance)

•Cannot control the urge of drinking when the effect of alcohol is wearing off; if not drinking, symptoms of alcohol withdrawal (nausea, sweating, anxiety, depression, trouble falling asleep, etc.) may be observed

•Cannot stop drinking even if the effects include getting a horrible hangover, being sick, missing workdays, and having family trouble (this indicates alcohol dependence)

•Cannot stop drinking even when aware of severe work-related (possibility of/or being fired from job due to drinking) and social problems

•More than once getting into trouble for drinking, for example, being prosecuted for DWI and being convicted, getting in trouble at work, and problems operating heavy machinery

If any of these symptoms or any other indications exist that indicate that a person is drinking in excess, medical intervention is very strongly recommended as the earlier the person seeks treatment, there is a very good chance of being cured. Many individuals with AUD have successfully completed alcohol rehabilitation treatment (outpatient or residential treatment) and live a normal healthy life.

It is important to know that the adverse effects of alcohol are not only associated with alcohol abuse and/or alcohol dependence (AUD), but also with heavy consumption of alcohol for a prolonged period of time regardless whether the person becomes alcohol dependent. For good health, it is advisable to follow the guidelines of the moderate consumption of alcohol. The health hazards of heavy alcohol consumption are listed in table 2.

Table 2. Adverse effects of heavy consumption of alcohol

Adverse outcome of heavy drinking	Comments
Fatty liver disease	Although moderate drinking (1.5 drinks or less per day), protects from fatty liver diseases, consumption of 3 or more drinks per day may increase the risk of fatty liver diseases. Another study indicated that above a threshold of 7-13 drinks per week for women, and 14-27 drinks per week for men, the risk of developing some alcohol-related liver disease was increased significantly.
Cirrhosis of the liver	A lifetime ingestion of 100 kg of alcohol (average of 3.9 drinks a day for approximately 5 years) is needed to develop cirrhosis of the liver. However, this disease may be potentially fatal.
Brain damage in adolescents	Early onset of drinking around age 13 has a devastating effect on the developing brain that may persist a lifetime. Teenagers and young adults below the age of 21 should not drink at all. Girls are more susceptible than boys.
Brain damage in adults	Smaller brain volume will result in both men and women with mental impairment and cognitive difficulties. However, women are affected more than men.
Korsakoff syndrome	This disease is observed in alcoholics mainly due to thiamine (vitamin B1) deficiency. Severe dementia is the major observation but abstinence from alcohol and proper treatment may be able to reverse some symptoms.
Wernicke-Korsakoff syndrome	In addition to dementia and confusion, visual problems and muscle weakness (e.g., difficulty walking) are also observed. Thiamine deficiency is the major cause of this disease.

Increased risk of cardiovascular diseases including heart attacks and heart failure	Consuming more than 3 drinks each day on a regular basis may cause some damage to the heart. Heavy drinking is also associated with hypertension, heart failure, alcoholic cardiomyopathy, and an increased risk of death after heart attack. Women are more susceptible to alcohol-induced heart damage than men.
Increased risk of stroke	Consuming 21 or more drinks weekly on a regular basis increases the risk of stroke, especially hemorrhagic stroke.
Increased risk of cancer	Excessive alcohol consumption is associated with cancer of the mouth, pharynx, larynx, and esophagus. Alcoholics may develop cirrhosis of the liver which may progress to liver cancer. Consuming 6 -11 drinks per day for 10-15 years may cause pancreatic cancer, a potential fatal disease.
Damage to the immune system	Alcohol reduces immunity and as result individuals consuming excessive amount of alcohol are more prone to both viral and bacterial infections.
Progression of AIDS	Even consuming 2 or more drinks per day on a regular basis may harm a patient despite receiving treatment.
Damage to endocrine system	A high alcohol concentration in the blood may interfere with the proper secretion of hormones from endocrine glands. Pseudo-Cushing's disease, which has all of the symptoms of Cushing's disease, may be observed in alcoholics.
Impaired fertility	Alcohol abuse is associated with fertility problems in both men and women.
Bone damage	Heavy consumption of alcohol may reduce bone mass thus increasing the risk of fractures after falls.
Fetal alcohol spectrum disorders and fetal alcohol syndrome	Pregnant women and women planning to be pregnant should not consume any alcohol.

Weight gain	Heavy alcohol consumption (over 30 gm a day, more than 2 drinks) is associated with significant weight gain.
Mood disorder, anxiety, and depression	Alcohol abuse is associated with mood disorders and major depression in both young adults and the elderly. Alcohol abuse may also increase the risk of late-life suicide.
Violent behavior	Alcohol abuse may cause aggressiveness and violent behavior. According to the U.S. Bureau of Justice, approximately 37% of state prison inmates and 21% of federal prison inmates serving time for violent crimes, were under the influence of alcohol when they committed crimes.
Reduced life span	Consuming alcohol exceeding the upper limit of moderate drinking and especially binge drinking may reduce life spans. People drinking 9 or more drinks on one occasion have a high risk of death following injury after binge drinking episodes.

Association of Liver Diseases Including Cirrhosis of the Liver with Heavy Drinking

If alcohol is consumed in moderation, the liver is effective in eliminating alcohol from the body by converting alcohol first to acetaldehyde by the action of alcohol dehydrogenase, and then by further converting acetaldehyde to acetate by the action of aldehyde dehydrogenase. Acetate is then converted into carbon dioxide and water. However, alcohol is toxic to the liver if the blood alcohol concentration is high. This is mainly due to the metabolism of alcohol by another liver enzyme, CYP2E1, which produces oxygen free radicals during the conversion of alcohol into acetaldehyde. These oxygen free radicals (increased oxidative stress) not only damage the liver but also damage other organs including the heart. Acetaldehyde, the metabolite of alcohol, is also toxic to the liver. In addition, alcohol consumption can potentiate other liver diseases such as hepatitis and non-alcoholic fatty liver diseases. Women are more susceptible to alcohol-related liver damage than men.

Although moderate alcohol consumption protects from fatty liver diseases, heavy alcohol consumption is associated with fatty changes in the liver. Kachele et al. (2015) (reported that the presence of a fatty liver was significantly reduced in subjects drinking 0-20 gm of alcohol per day (up to 1.5 drinks a day) compared to people drinking 40-60 gm (3 to 4 drinks) of alcohol per day (6). Heavy drinking for as little as a few days, may produce fatty changes in the liver (steatosis) which is reversed after abstinence. Steatosis may be present in 90% of heavy drinkers. However, drinking heavily for a longer period may cause more severe alcohol-related liver injuries such as alcoholic hepatitis which, with continued heavy alcohol consumption, may progress to cirrhosis of the liver.

The amount of alcohol consumed is one of the determining factors in developing alcoholic hepatitis and eventually cirrhosis of the liver. In one report the authors commented that cirrhosis of the liver does not develop below a lifetime ingestion of 100 kg of alcohol (1 standard drink is approximately 14 gm of alcohol; therefore a lifetime consumption of 7,143 drinks). This amount corresponds to an average of 3.9 drinks a day for approximately 5 years. The authors also commented that consuming alcohol with food lowers the risk of developing cirrhosis of the liver if alcohol is consumed on an empty stomach (7). In general, it is considered that the threshold of alcohol-induced liver toxicity is 40 gm of alcohol per day (approximately 3 drinks a day) for men, and 30 gm (more than just 2 drinks) or more alcohol a day for women over a period of 5 years. The highest risk is associated with consuming 8.6 drinks (120 gm of alcohol) per day (8). However, another study indicated that above a threshold of 7-13 drinks per week for women, and 14-27 drinks per week for men, the risk for developing some alcohol- related liver diseases was increased significantly. The greater sensitivity of women toward alcohol toxicity may be related to the genetic predisposition of the metabolism pattern of alcohol in women where more oxidative byproducts of alcohol are formed compared to men. Consumption of coffee may protect males against alcohol-induced liver damage but no such data is currently available for females (9).

Hepatitis C is a liver disease caused by the hepatitis C virus. Alcohol consumption potentiates hepatitis C infection. Whether a person with this infection can drink in moderation is an open question. In one study the authors observed that moderate alcohol consumption between 31 and50 gm per day (approximately 2 to 3 1/2 drinks) for males, and 21-50 gm per day (1 1/2 to 3 1/2 drinks) for females could adversely affect the progression of liver damage (10). If you are diagnosed with hepatitis C infection do not consume any amount of alcohol without consultation with your physician. Fortunately, there are new treatment options available for hepatitis C which are very effective and even curative.

Alcohol-Related Brain Damage

Although alcohol can cause relaxation and mild euphoria with moderate consumption; these pleasurable effects disappear with increasing blood alcohol levels. Alcohol has more damaging effects on the adolescence brain than on the adult brain. Onset of drinking at an early age (13 or earlier) has devastating effects on the developing brain and such adverse effects (neurocognitive deficiency, e.g., learning disability, poor memory, and other impairment of brain function) may persist a lifetime. The early onset of drinking is also linked to greater risks of alcohol dependence in adult life. Underage drinkers are also susceptible to the immediate ill effects of alcohol use such as blackouts, hangovers, and alcohol poisoning.

Women are more susceptible to alcohol-related

neurological damage than men, in particular, the female adolescent brain is more vulnerable to alcohol exposure than a male adolescent brain. Adolescents with alcohol abuse disorders have smaller prefrontal cortex brain volumes compared to healthy adolescents. The prefrontal cortex located in the frontal lobe of the brain is a crucial area of the brain responsible for planning complex cognitive behavior such as learning, critical thinking, working with information held mentally, rational judgment, expression of personality, and appropriate social behavior. Alcohol use during adolescence is associated with lower prefrontal volume but girls are more affected than boys (11).

The two major alcohol-related brain damages are alcoholic Korsakoff's syndrome and alcoholic dementia. Korsakoff's syndrome is a brain disorder caused by a deficiency of thiamine (vitamin B1) and symptoms are severe memory loss, lack of insight, poor conversation skills, and apathy (12). When Wernicke's encephalopathy accompanies Korsakoff's syndrome in an alcoholic, it is called Wernicke-Korsakoff syndrome. Wernicke's encephalopathy and Korsakoff's syndrome are two related diseases, both caused by thiamine deficiency. Alcoholics with only Korsakoff's syndrome always have severe amnesic syndromes but may not have classical symptoms of Wernicke's encephalopathy which include ophthalmoplegia (paralysis or weakness of eye muscles causing double vision, blurred vision, and other problems), ataxia (lack of muscle control causing difficulty in walking, picking up objects, etc.), and confusion. The Royal College of Physicians in London recommends that patients admitted to the hospital who show evidence of the chronic misuse of alcohol and poor diet should be treated with B vitamins (13). Other than developing Korsakoff's syndrome or Wernicke-Korsakoff syndrome, thiamine deficiency in chronic alcohol abusers is a major cause of alcohol-induced brain damage.

Chronic abuse of alcohol results in brain damage to both males and females but women are more susceptible to alcohol-induced brain damage than men. In general, reduction of brain volume including the volume of gray and white matter is observed in both alcoholic men and women compared to the brain volume of moderate drinkers and teetotalers. However, the difference between brain volume in a healthy woman and in an alcoholic woman is more significant than the difference in brain volume between a healthy man and an alcoholic man. Binge drinkers, both males and females, are at higher risks of developing alcohol-related brain damage.

Alcohol-related brain damage and loss of cognitive functions may be reversible at least in part, if the brain damage is not permanent and if the alcoholics can successfully complete a rehabilitation program and practice complete abstinence. Chronic alcoholism is often associated with brain shrinkage but this may be reversed at least in part when abstinence is maintained as demonstrated by Trabert et al. (1995), based on a study using 28 male patients with severe alcohol dependence. Even with three weeks of abstinence, densities of brain tissues were increased in these subjects (14).

Increased Risk of Cardiovascular Diseases and Stroke Due to Heavy Drinking

Although moderate alcohol consumption is associated with a reduced risk of cardiovascular disease, people who consume excess alcohol have higher risks of cardiovascular diseases including myocardial infarction, cardiomyopathy, and heart failure. Even drinking more than 3alcoholic beverages regularly may have an adverse effect on the heart including disturbances of heart rhythm. Heavy drinking is associated with increased blood pressure (hypertension) which is harmful to the heart and which may increase the risk of stroke. Alcoholics who consume 90 gm or more of alcohol a day (7drinks) for five years are at a very high risk of developing alcoholic cardiomyopathy and if they continue drinking alcohol, cardiomyopathy may proceed to heart failure, a potentially fatal condition. Without complete abstinence, 50% of these patients may die within the next four years of developing heart failure (15). Women are at a higher risk of alcoholic cardiomyopathy than men. Chronic consumption of excess alcohol is also associated with a higher risk of death after a heart attack (16). Heavy drinking also increases the risk of stroke, particularly the risk of hemorrhagic stroke. In one study, the authors observed that the risk of hemorrhagic stroke increases in an individual drinking 300 gm or more of alcohol weekly (21 or more drinks weekly) (17).

Heavy Alcohol Consumption Increases the Risk of Certain Cancers

There is a relation between consumption of excessive amounts of alcohol and developing certain types of cancers. The strongest link was found between alcohol abuse and cancer of the mouth, pharynx, larynx, and esophagus. An estimated 75% of all esophageal cancers are attributable to chronic alcohol abuse while nearly 50% of cancers of the mouth, pharynx, and larynx are associated with chronic heavy consumption of alcohol. Prolonged drinking may result in alcoholic liver disease and cirrhosis of the liver and such diseases can progress to liver carcinoma (liver cancer). Heavy consumption of alcohol (80-150 gm, approximately 6 -11 drinks per day) for 10-15 years may cause pancreatic cancer. Although a small percentage of alcoholics (2-5%), may eventually develop pancreatic cancer, this disease is potentially fatal. Pancreatitis may occur in alcoholics due to the consumption of excessive amounts of alcohol on a daily basis.

The relation between moderate alcohol consumption and the risk of breast cancer is controversial because there are conflicting reports in the medical literature. One Spanish study using 762 women between 18 and 75 years of age showed that women who consumed 20 gm or more alcohol a day (1 1/2 drinks or more) have a higher chance of developing breast cancer than nondrinkers (18). In contrast, another study reported that women who consumed 10 to 12 gm wine per day (1 glass of wine) had a lower risk of developing breast cancer compared to nondrinkers. However, the risk of breast cancer increases in women who consumed more than 1drink per day (19). Nagata et al. (2007), based on a review of 11 reports on the association between alcohol consumption and the risk of breast cancer, concluded that epidemiological evidence of the link between moderate alcohol consumption and the risk of developing breast cancer remains insufficient. However, drinking 23 gm or more alcohol (1 1/2 drinks) per day may significantly increase the risk of breast cancer (20). Pelucchi et al. (2011) concluded that the consumption of fewer than 3 alcoholic drinks per week is not associated with an increased risk of breast cancer, but consuming 3 to 6 drinks per week may be associated with a small increase in risk (21).

Heavy Alcohol Consumption and Damage to the Immune System

Alcohol abuse is associated with an increased risk of bacterial and viral infection due to impairment of the immune system. Mast cells are important immune cells which are widely distributed in tissues and are also in contact with the external environment such as skin, mucosa of the lungs, and the gastrointestinal tract. Mast cells produce a variety of compounds which play important roles in the defense against bacteria and parasite. Alcohol reduces the viability of mast cells and may cause cell death. As a result, alcohol-induced reduction of the viability of mast cells could contribute to an impaired immune system associated with alcohol abuse. Alcohol also accelerates disease progression in patients with HIV infection due to impairment of the immune system. In one study using 231 patients with HIV infection who were undergoing antiretroviral therapy, the authors observed that even consumption of 2 or more drinks daily can cause a serious decline in CD4+ cell count (lower CD4+ counts indicates a progression of AIDS) (22).

Heavy Alcohol Consumption and Damage to Endocrine System, Reproductive System, and Bones

Alcohol abuse can have adverse effects on the human endocrine system because alcohol in high concentrations may reduce the secretion of various hormones essential for life. Alcohol abuse may lead to a disease known as pseudo Cushings syndrome which is indistinguishable from Cushings syndrome and is characterized by the excess production of cortisol (stress hormone). As a result, high blood pressure, muscle weakness, diabetes, obesity, and a variety of other physical disturbances may occur in an individual consuming an excess amount of alcohol.

Diminished sexual function in alcoholic men has been described for many years. Administration of alcohol in healthy young male volunteers caused diminished levels of testosterone. Excessive alcohol consumption (more than 60 gm a day, more than 4 drinks) is strongly associated with azoospermia (lack of any viable sperm in the semen causing infertility). Guthauser et al. (2014) reported the case of a man who had azoospermia due to alcohol abuse but was able to father a child following assisted reproduction technique two years after complete withdrawal from alcohol (23). Even drinking 3 or more drinks a day may cause significant problems in women including delayed ovulation or failure to ovulate, and menstrual problems but such problems were not noticed in women who consumed 2 or fewer drinks a day. Alcoholic women often experience reproductive problems. However, these problems may be resolved when a woman practices abstinence from alcohol.

To form healthy bone calcium, phosphorus and an active form of vitamin D is essential. Chronic consumption of alcohol may reduce bone mass through a complex process of inhibition of hormonal balance needed for bone growth including testosterone in men which is diminished in alcoholics. Alcohol abuse may also interfere with pancreatic secretion of insulin causing diabetes (24).

Fetal Alcohol Disorders and Fetal Alcohol Syndrome

As mentioned in chapter 2, pregnant women and women planning to be pregnant should not drink at all. Fetal alcohol spectrum disorders and fetal alcohol syndrome are related diseases both caused by maternal drinking during pregnancy. Fetal alcohol syndrome is the more severe form of the disease. Maternal alcohol consumption significantly increases the risk of miscarriage and stillbirth. If the newborn survives, the child may face mental retardation, learning difficulties and development problems for the rest of their lives. Based on a review of available medical literature, May and Gossage (2001) estimated that the prevalence of fetal alcohol syndrome in the United States is 0.5 to 2.0 cases per 1,000 births (25).

Heavy Alcohol Consumption Associated with Mood Disorder and Depression

Alcohol can provide stress relief if consumed in moderation, but with higher blood alcohol, alcohol acts as a central nervous system depressant, which is responsible for many ill effects of alcohol at high blood alcohol concentration. Heavy alcohol consumption is associated with anxiety and depression. One of the reasons for alcoholic hangovers is the presence of acetaldehyde, the major metabolite of alcohol. However, high anxiety among college students may cause alcohol abuse after social interaction. Many college students also consume excessive amounts of alcohol to combat stress, but in reality, alcohol abuse increases stress and anxiety. Several studies also demonstrated that alcohol-induced major depression in young adults. Blow et al. (2014) observed that alcohol abuse was also associated with depression in the elderly and may increase the risk of late life suicide (26).

Alcohol Abuse and Violent Behavior/Crime

Many investigators reported a close link between violent behavior, homicide, and alcohol intoxication. Studies conducted on convicted murders suggested that about half of them were under the heavy influence of alcohol at the time of murder (27). Alcohol may induce aggression and violent behavior by disrupting normal brain function when consumed in high dosages. By impairing the normal information -processing capability of the brain, a person can misjudge a perceived threat and may react more aggressively than warranted. Serotonin, a neurotransmitter, is considered a behavioral inhibitor. Alcohol abuse may lead to decreased serotonin activity causing aggressive behavior. Alcohol abuse by the husband may be related to marital violence. Studies have shown the link between alcohol abuse by the husband before marriage, and husband to wife aggression in the first year of marriage. The violence occurs more frequently when the husband was a heavy drinker and the wife was not (28). According to the U.S. Bureau of Justice, approximately 37% of state prison inmates and 21% of federal prison inmates serving time for violent crimes, were under the influence of alcohol when they committed crimes.

Alcohol Abuse and Reduced Life Span

Although moderate drinking is associated with increased longevity, alcohol abuse is associated with decreased longevity compared to abstainers. Even occasional heavy drinking may be detrimental to health. Dawson (2001) reported an increased risk of mortality among individuals who consumed alcohol less than once a month but were binge drinkers (drinking more than 5 drinks in one occasion) (29). In a British study, the authors, based on an investigation of 5,766 men aged 35-64 with 21 years of follow-up, observed that men who consumed over 15 standard alcoholic beverages per week, had significantly higher risks of dying from all causes compared to nondrinkers. In addition, individuals who consumed over

35 drinks per week, had double the risk of mortality compared to nondrinkers (30). The London-based Whitehall II cohort study using 10,308 government employees between the ages of 35 and 55, with 11-year follow-ups, concluded that optimal drinking is the daily consumption of 1drink or less once or twice a week. People who consumed more had an increased risk of mortality compared to those drinking once or twice a week (31).

Binge drinking is also dangerous because one study based on 13,251 adults who reported binge drinking, concluded that death due to injuries were significantly elevated compared to persons who drank fewer than 5drinks in a single occasion. Persons dinking 9 or more drinks in a single occasion had even a much higher risk to die from injuries than people consuming less than 5drinks (32). Other than increasing mortality from various diseases, alcohol abuse is also associated with an increased risk of suicide, accidents, and violent crimes. Based on a survey of 31,953 high school students, Schilling et al. (2009) observed that both drinking while depressed and episodic heavy drinking were associated with self-reported suicide attempts in adolescents (33).

Alcohol Poisoning

Drinking excessive alcohol on one occasion may cause alcohol poisoning which if not treated promptly, may be fatal. In general, alcohol poisoning occurs at a blood alcohol level of 0.3% and above, but significant alcohol toxicity may be observed at much lower blood alcohol concentrations in some individuals. If a man weighing 150 pounds consumes 11 drinks in one hour, the calculated blood alcohol is 0.31%, using the Widmark formula. Kanny et al. (reported that alcohol poisoning typically occurs following binge drinking. An annual average of death from alcohol poisoning, based on a review of many reports, was 2,221 (8.8 deaths per 1 million) in persons age 15 years and older. Of these deaths, 1,681 (75.7%) involved adults age 35-64 years, and 1,696 were men. The authors concluded that on average 6 people, mostly adult men, die from alcohol poisoning each day in the United States (34). Alcohol poisoning is a medical emergency and immediate treatment in a medical facility is needed to avoid fatalities.

Dangers of Mixing Alcohol with Drug Abuse

Alcohol is often abused with illicit drugs and such practices may cause serious drug toxicity and even fatality. The simultaneous abuse of cocaine and alcohol may cause serious toxicity and death due to the formation of "cocaethylene," a lethal metabolite of cocaine which is only formed in the presence of alcohol. Alcohol also significantly reduces the toxicity threshold of many benzodiazepines and opioid pain medication. Sometimes addicts crush extended release oxycodone tablets to form powder or to dissolve it in a solvent and then ingest it. Extended release tablets are prepared in such a way that only a small amount of oxycodone is released at a given time so that oxycodone is present in the blood for a prolonged time up to 12 hours. Crushing such tablets may result in oxycodone overdose which may even be fatal.

Dangers of Drinking Moonshine Whiskey

The current U. S. laws permit the home production of beer and wine by fermentation for personal use. However, the sale of such alcoholic beverages is not permitted, and federal law does not permit the production of distilled liquor such as whiskey because if not done properly, it may cause harm. Moonshine liquors are defined as any illegally produced alcohol worldwide. Because such products are not prepared using rigorous technical processes, harmful compounds such as lead and heavy metals may be present in moonshine whiskey. As a result, lead poisoning may occur after drinking moonshine whiskey for a few weeks. Although uncommon in the United States, in developing countries methanol (which is inexpensive) is added to moonshine whiskey and consuming such alcohol may cause blindness and even death. The *New York Times* on May 21, 2008, reported the death of 110 people in Bangalore, India, in nearby rural areas, and across the state border of Tamil Nadu after the consumption of illegally produced liquor.

Dangers of Drinking Methanol and Ethylene Glycol

Denatured alcohol (methylated spirit) is inexpensive and contains mostly ethanol (alcohol) and 10% methanol. Sometimes isopropyl alcohol, acetone, methyl ethyl ketone, and so forth, are also added to produce a bitter taste so that this liquid in undrinkable. Methanol is a toxic chemical which if consumed, may cause blindness and even fatality. Ethylene glycol is found in antifreeze and is also used in the radiator fluid (along with fluorescein so that during radiator leaks, a motor mechanic can identify the leak due to the fluorescence property of this compound). This product must be kept out of reach of children and pets because it has a sweet taste. A dog may die after drinking a small amount of ethylene glycol due to kidney failure. A human may also die after abusing ethylene glycol due to kidney failure.

Conclusions

Heavy drinking on a regular basis may lead to alcohol use disorder. The major complication of excessive alcohol consumption is alcohol-induced liver damage where women are more susceptible than men. Moreover, underage drinking is associated with alcohol-induced brain damage that may affect the person throughout their lives. According to the report of the National Institute of Alcohol Abuse and Alcoholism, nearly 88,000 people (approximately 62,000 men and 26,000 women) die from alcohol-related causes in the United States each year, making alcohol-related deaths the fourth leading preventable cause of deaths. Therefore, the best practice is to follow the guidelines of moderate drinking and to enjoy the many health benefits of alcohol.

However, consuming alcohol in excess is a health hazard. The good news is that alcohol use disorder is a psychiatric illness and with proper medical care, alcohol abuse as well as alcohol use disorder can be completely cured. There are medications for treating alcohol abuse. If you know any friend or loved one who may be consuming too much alcohol, make sure that they get medical attention as soon as possible. Some alcohol-related damage to the human body may be partly or fully reversible.

5 ENVIRONMENTAL AND GENETIC FACTORS LINKED TO DRINKING

Introduction

Many factors are associated with the susceptibility of a person to alcohol abuse. In general, more men than women abuse alcohol. Unfortunately, women are also more susceptible to alcohol- related adverse health effects. Although family studies have shown that the risk for alcohol abuse is 4 to 10 fold higher in an offspring of an alcoholic parent, it is important to remember that alcohol abuse is not a totally inheritable genetic disorder. Inherited disorders, for example, familial hypercholesterolemia (when a genetic defect may increase serum cholesterol to 500 to 1,000 mg/dL where the desirable normal level is below 200 mg/dL), Huntington's disease, sickle cell anemia, cystic fibrosis, Tay-Sachs disease, phenylketonuria, hemophilia, and so forth, are inheritable genetic disorders where one particular defective gene is involved with each disorder. However, there is no single gene that causes alcohol use disorder.

In general, it is assumed that genetic factors may contribute 50%, while environmental factors contribute another 50% in developing the susceptibility of an individual for alcohol abuse. The legal age of drinking in the United States is 21; and parents must ensure that their adolescent children should not consume any alcohol. Underage drinking is not only associated with poor performance in school, but is also associated with an increased risk of abusing alcohol. Moreover, underage drinking is harmful for the developing adolescent brain (see also chapter 4).

Environmental Factors in Childhood and in Adolescence

Environmental factors of childhood play important roles in the proper physical and emotional development of the child. Childhood neglect or abuse is a major risk factor that is linked to underage drinking. Peer pressure experienced by teenagers in the school environment also contributes significantly in their first underage experiment with alcohol. Prenatal exposure of alcohol is associated with a higher likelihood of the child to abuse alcohol or to other substances during adolescent years. Tomcikova et al. (2015), based on a study sample of 3,882 individuals, concluded that living with one parent is associated with an increased risk of frequent drinking and drunkenness among adolescents. Moreover, a low quality of communication between mother and child is associated with an increased risk of adolescent drinking (1). Having strict parental rules for not drinking is associated with minimum or no alcohol use by the adolescents. However, parents' permissiveness toward drinking is associated with a higher frequency of alcohol consumption by adolescents (2).

Physical abuse (involving mostly male children) and sexual abuse (involving mostly female children) during childhood is associated with a higher risk of adolescent alcohol or drug abuse. Many studies have shown that physical and sexual abuse may predict later alcohol and drug abuse. Skinner et al. (2016) followed 332 participants from childhood (18 months to 6 years of age) to adulthood (31-41 years of age) and observed that childhood sexual abuse was fully mediated by alcohol use and by depression into their adolescent years and also into their mid-30s (3). UNICEF has estimated that between 133 and275 million children around the world witness frequent parental conflict or violence. Smith et al. (2010) concluded that exposure to severe intimate partner violence as an adolescent significantly increased the odds of alcohol use problems in early adulthood for young women but not for young men (4). Bullying or being a victim of bullying may increase the risk of alcohol use in high school. High school students who are affiliated with gangs are more likely to abuse alcohol and drugs.

A positive environment in childhood and during the adolescence years protect an individual from drinking or from experimenting with drugs. Studies have shown that parental supervision and monitoring resulted in lower alcohol or substance abuse among 8th and 10th graders. Moreover, good grades in school and having peers who do not drink is associated with low or no alcohol use in high school. When these individuals graduate from high school and attend college, if roommates and peers do not consume alcohol, these individuals also refrain from drinking. Various risk factors for adolescent alcohol and environmental factors that protect from alcohol use are summarized in table 1.

Table 1. Childhood and adolescence environment and underage drinking

Environmental factors that increase the risk of alcohol use	**Environmental factors that protect from alcohol use**
Drinking during pregnancy increases the risk of offspring to abuse alcohol.	Parents are married and living together, good communication between mother and child, and a close relationship with parents have protective effects.
Risk for alcohol abuse is 4 to	Strict parental rules against

10 fold higher in the offspring of an alcoholic parent. However, the offspring of an alcoholic parent can also be a teetotaler because there is no single gene related to alcoholism.	drinking and close monitoring of child/adolescent have a protecting effect.
Young adults living with one parent have a higher risk of alcohol use.	Good academic performance and good grades in school have a protective effect.
Childhood maltreatment and physical or sexual abuse may increase the risk of underage drinking.	Parents not drinking at all or drinking in moderation also have protective effects.
Intimate partner conflict/violence usually increases the risk of the alcoholic abuse of the female child when she reaches adolescence or adulthood.	Peers in school who do not drink protect an adolescent from drinking.
Bullying increases the risk of alcohol use for both the bully and the victim.	Roommates in college not drinking and peers in college not drinking also protect a college student from drinking.
Joining a gang in high school increases the risk of alcohol and substance abuse.	Religious affiliations of parents, religiosity, and spirituality also have protective effects.
Parents have a casual view of underage drinking and there is easy availability of alcohol in the household	
Poor mother-child communication may increase the risk of drinking when the child reaches adolescent years	

Stress May Increase Alcohol Consumption

The body responds to stress with self-regulating processes which contain both physiological and psychological components. In general, stress increases the production of cortisol, the stress hormone due to activation of hypothalamic-pituitary-adrenal axis (HPA-axis). A healthy acute stress response is characterized by a quick rise in blood cortisol level followed by a decline of cortisol level to the basal level with the termination of the stressful event. However, if a person is subjected to chronic stress, hypercortisolemia (elevated cortisol level) may occur. Many stressful events such as changing jobs; moving; trouble with a boss, coworker, neighbor, or family member; poor health; being a victim of a crime; being fired or unemployed; and divorce or breakup may increase a person's susceptibility to consume an excessive amount of alcohol.

Terrorist attacks may also increase alcohol use among people as studies have shown that following the terrorist attacks that destroyed the World Trade Center in New York in 2001, alcohol consumption was increased in New York City and elsewhere for a short period after the attack. Longer-term studies showed increased alcohol consumption 1 and 2 years later among New Yorkers who had greater exposure to the attack (5). Various life stressors that may increase susceptibility to alcohol abuse and environmental factors that may protect an adult from alcohol abuse are listed in table 2.

Table 2. Life stressors that increase the risk of heavy drinking in an adult and factors that protect from drinking

Life stressors that increase the risk of an adult to heavy drinking	Factors that protect and adult from heavy drinking
Being fired from a job	Married and spouse consumes alcohol in moderation or does not drink
Changing a job	Successful and happy work environment and having

	financial stability
Serious or life-threatening illnesses in family members/close friends	Close tie with family members
Serious financial trouble	Close tie with friends who either drink in moderation or do not drink.
Divorce or separation	Good social network
Living alone	Peers are moderate drinkers or do not drink
Difficulty with spouse/family member/children	Religiosity/spirituality protects from heavy drinking
Living in a neighborhood with a high crime rate	Practicing yoga and/or meditation
Legal trouble	

Marriage has a protective effect on alcohol or substance abuse. Kendler et al. (2016), based on a population study involving 3,220,628 individuals, concluded that first marriages to a spouse with no lifetime alcohol use disorder was associated with a large reduction in risk of alcohol use disorder. These observations are consistent with the hypothesis that the psychological and social aspects of marriage and in particular health-monitoring spousal interactions, strongly protect against the development of alcohol use disorder (6). Close ties with family members, a good social network, having peers and friends who do not abuse alcohol or drug and religiosity/spirituality are protective factors against the development of alcohol or drug use. The practice of yoga and meditation may have protective effects against alcohol or drug abuse. Reddy et al. (2014) concluded that a specialized yoga therapy may play a role in attenuating the symptoms of PTSD (posttraumatic stress disorder), reducing the risk of alcohol and drug use (7).

Certain Personality Types and Alcohol Use
The Five Factor Model of personality developed by

McCreae and John (1992) is one of the most commonly used models in psychology. The model consists of five personality factors which can be evaluated using the revised NEO Personality Inventory Facet Scale (8).

•Openness

•Conscientiousness

•Extraversion

•Agreeableness

•Neuroticism (negative emotions)

Martin and Sher (1994), based on a study of 468 young adults, observed that alcohol use disorder was positively associated with neuroticism and negatively associated with agreeableness and conscientiousness (9). Impulsivity is related to risk taking, quick decision making, and lack of planning. Such behavior is often committed in the spur of the moment without paying attention to consequences including negative effects. Impulsivity is closely linked to alcohol and substance abuse (10). Novelty-seeking behavior also increases the risk of alcohol abuse in a person. Again, alcohol and drug abuse is a psychiatric problem which can be reversed by proper medical treatments.

Genes and Alcohol Consumption

The human genome contains 3.2 billion nucleotides of DNA. The most common genetic mutation is single nucleotide polymorphism (where a single nucleotide that occurs in the specific position of the normal DNA structure is replaced by another nucleotide). As a result, an amino acid in the normal sequence of proteins is replaced by another amino acid. If the protein is an enzyme, that may alter normal enzymatic function (inactive of superactive enzymes). Although SNPs are the most common genetic variation, other variations including deletion, insertion, and duplication may also occur.

There are two strategies to identify genes related to the

vulnerability for alcohol dependence. One is genome-wide analysis and another is candidate gene association study. Alcohol is metabolized by alcohol and aldehyde dehydrogenase. Mutations of genes that encode these enzymes may significantly affect alcohol metabolism and may protect a person from alcohol consumption. Alcohol exerts its effects through various neurotransmitter systems in the brain. As a result, certain mutations of genes encoding such complex neurotransmitters systems may also play a role in determining the susceptibility of a person to alcohol abuse. Currently, mutations of genes that encode alcohol-metabolizing enzymes and their relationship with alcohol consumption are best understood. Many studies have also found an association between alcohol abuse and mutated genes involved in neural transmission (e.g., GABA, dopamine, and serotonin receptors) but results are inconsistent among various studies (11).

Mutations of Genes Encoding Alcohol-Metabolizing Enzymes and Protection from Alcohol Use

Alcohol is metabolized by alcohol dehydrogenase enzyme into acetaldehyde. Then acetaldehyde is converted into acetate by aldehyde dehydrogenase. Unpleasant reactions after consuming alcohol such as facial flushing, nausea, headaches, and rapid heartbeats known as alcohol flushing or alcohol intolerance, is due to acetaldehyde, the first metabolite of alcohol. Usually, acetaldehyde is not detected in the blood due to very low concentration but in individuals with alcohol intolerance, acetaldehyde may be detected in the blood. Alcohol intolerance is not an allergic reaction but is a condition which can only be avoided by not consuming alcohol. Usually this is observed more commonly in the Asian population but individuals belonging to other racial groups may also have alcohol intolerance.

Alcohol flushing reaction and alcohol intolerance may deter an individual from drinking. This is may be caused by mutations in the gene that encodes aldehyde dehydrogenase enzymes. These mutations are single nucleotide polymorphisms. The aldehyde dehydrogenase enzyme encoded by a defective gene usually has poor enzymatic activity. As a result, acetaldehyde is not efficiently removed from the blood causing acetaldehyde buildup and an unpleasant reaction from drinking. Another cause is genetic mutation that encodes superactive alcohol dehydrogenase enzyme. Therefore, alcohol is quickly metabolized to acetaldehyde causing acetaldehyde buildup in the blood because even normally active aldehyde dehydrogenase cannot remove such high amounts of acetaldehyde fast enough. Individuals with this genetic mutation also consume alcohol to avoid unpleasant reactions after drinking.

The aldehyde dehydrogenase enzyme (ALDH2) responsible for the metabolism of acetaldehyde is encoded by *ALDH2* gene. The most common genetic mutations (polymorphism) is *ALDH2*2* genetic allele that encodes the poorly active ALDH2 enzyme thus protecting an individual from alcohol abuse due to acetaldehyde buildup. This mutation is found among 45% of East Asians including Han Chinese, Japanese, and Koreans but rarely in other ethnic groups. It has been estimated that 540 million people worldwide (8% of the world population) carry this genetic mutation. Homozygous genetic mutation produces inactive enzymes but heterozygous genetic mutations may have partial enzymatic activity. Genetic and epidemiological studies have shown that homozygous individuals are almost fully protected from drinking alcohol but heterozygous individuals have partial protection (approximately 60%) from alcohol abuse (12).

The class I alcohol dehydrogenase enzymes (ADH) responsible for the majority of the metabolism of alcohol into acetaldehyde are encoded by *ADH1A, ADH1B,* and *ADH1C* genes. There are two superactive ADH enzymes due to polymorphisms of genes encoding ADH enzyme.

One such polymorphism is the *ADH1B*2* gene which is found commonly among East Asians (Han Chinese, Japanese, Koreans, Filipinos, Malays, etc. and aborigines of Australia and New Zealand) and also among approximately 25% of people of Jewish origin. This genetic mutation is also encountered in small frequency among Caucasians. ADH enzymes encoded by this mutated gene are superactive, causing the rapid metabolism of alcohol into acetaldehyde and acetaldehyde buildup in the blood. This deters an individual carrying this genetic mutation from consuming alcohol. Although *ADH1B*2* is more prevalent in Asians and protects these individuals from alcohol abuse, if this mutation is present in Caucasians, it has the same effect (13). Carr et al. (2002) reported that men in the *ADH1B*2* allele group reported more unpleasant reactions to alcohol compared to men carrying the wild type (unmutated) gene (14).

Both *ALDH2*2* and ADH1B*2 genetic mutations have protective effects against alcohol abuse. Sometimes both genetic mutations are present in one person and usually that provides 100% protection; the person is usually a teetotaler. There are also other genetic mutations that have protective effects against alcohol abuse. Genetic mutations that protect against alcohol abuse are summarized in table 3.

Table 3. Common mutations of genes that protect from alcohol abuse

Mutation of the gene	Enzymatic activity	Cause of protection from alcohol use
ALDH2*2	Poor enzymatic activity of aldehyde dehydrogenase	Unpleasant reaction after drinking due to acetaldehyde buildup (slow removal of acetaldehyde due to poor enzymatic activity)
ADH1B*2	Superactive alcohol dehydrogenase	Fast metabolism of alcohol into acetaldehyde which

		causes acetaldehyde buildup despite normally active aldehyde dehydrogenase enzymes
ALDH2*2 and ADH1B*2	Poorly active aldehyde dehydrogenase but superactive active alcohol dehydrogenase	Significant acetaldehyde buildup giving complete protection from using alcohol
ADH1B*3	Superactive active alcohol dehydrogenase	Protection from alcohol abuse due to acetaldehyde buildup

Although certain mutations in genes encoding alcohol and aldehyde dehydrogenase are implicated in protecting individuals against alcohol abuse, there is no evidence that people with normally functioning alcohol and aldehyde dehydrogenase enzymes may be susceptible to consuming too much alcohol. Most people who consume alcohol in moderation have normally functioning alcohol-metabolizing enzymes.

Other Genes Related to Alcohol Abuse

Interestingly, alcohol and drug abuse are related to each other because many neurological pathways delivering rewards after drinking alcohol are also associated with drug-induced euphoria. The central function of the human brain is due to the presence of 100 billion neurons and everything humans do relies on communications between neurons. Synapses are small gaps between neurons where messages move from one neuron to another neuron mostly as a chemical signal via neurotransmitters. More than 180 neurotransmitters have been described but common neurotransmitters are dopamine, serotonin GABA (gamma-aminobutyric acid), epinephrine, norepinephrine glutamate, and acetylcholine. Neurotransmitters can be divided under two broad groups, inhibitory or excitatory. Excitatory neurotransmitters stimulate neurons and the brain while inhibitory neurotransmitters have a calming effect, but some neurotransmitters may play a dual role. As mentioned earlier in this chapter, the mutations of genes encoding various neurotransmitter pathways and their association with alcohol abuse are not clearly understood due to conflicting reports in the medical literature.

In general, GABA inhibitory neurotransmission is considered to mediate pleasurable effects in the brain after drinking. GABA receptors are proteins encoded by various genes and mutations of *GABR2* genes that encode GABA-A receptors may increase the risk of alcohol abuse. Other mutations in genes encoding various GABA receptors may also be linked with alcohol abuse. Mutations of genes (*CHRM2*) encoding the cholinergic muscarinic receptor-2 may also be related to alcohol dependence. Mutations of certain genes encoding opioid receptors, dopamine receptors, and dopamine and serotonin transporters are also associated with alcohol dependence. An in-depth discussion on this very complex topic is beyond the scope of this book.

Conclusions

Some environmental factors increase the susceptibility of a person for alcohol abuse while other environmental factors protect against alcohol abuse. Many life stressors may also increase the vulnerability of an individual for alcohol abuse but effective stress control though family networks, friends, peers, and one's spouse can alleviate the negative effects of stress. Certain mutations of genes encoding alcohol and aldehyde dehydrogenase have protective effects against alcohol abuse. However, genetic inheritance of alcohol dependence can be counterbalances by positive environmental factors. Therefore, unlike genetic diseases that are transmitted from parents to offspring, alcohol dependence is not a genetic disease although there may be a genetic component. No single gene has been identified that is related to alcohol abuse. The good news is that although the risk of the offspring of alcoholic parents becoming alcohol dependent in the later part of life is higher than the risk of offspring of non-alcoholic parents, this risk can be counterbalanced by environmental factors and it is absolutely possible that children of alcoholic parents are teetotalers when they reach adulthood.

6 BEER, WINE, OR VODKA: WHAT SHOULD I DRINK?

Introduction

Consuming alcohol in moderation (up to 2 drinks a day for a man, and up to 1 drink a day for a woman) has many health benefits including reduced risk of cardiovascular diseases (including heart attacks), stroke, cancer (certain types), type 2 diabetes, arthritis, and gallstones as well as increased longevity. Although many health benefits of drinking in moderation are attributable to the alcohol content of alcoholic beverages, not all benefits are due to alcohol alone. Beer, wine, and cocktails (coming from fruits/fruit juice) contain many beneficial polyphenols and phenolic compounds which act as antioxidants. In addition, these compounds have many other beneficial effects on health. The comparison of beer, wine, and spirit for their beneficial effects on health are given in table 1.

Table 1. Comparison of beer, wine, and spirits for various health benefits associated with moderate consumption of alcoholic beverages

Health benefit	Beer	Wine	Sprit	Comments
Reduced overall risk of	++	++	+	Although drinking any alcoholic

cardiovascular disease				beverages is good for a healthy heart, beer and wine seems to be superior to sprits due to the presence of polyphenolic compounds. Maybe red wine is slightly superior.
Increased concentration of good cholesterol (HDL-cholesterol)	++	++	++	Alcohol is responsible for increasing the concentration of good cholesterol in the blood.
Reduced risk of ischemic stroke	++	++	++	Consuming any alcoholic beverage is associated with a decreased risk.
Reduced risk of Type 2 diabetes	++	++	++	Consuming any alcoholic beverage is associated with a decreased risk.
Protection from certain types of cancer	+	++		Polyphenolic compounds present in beer and wine may reduce the risk, but wine is more effective.
Reduced risk of rheumatoid arthritis	++	++	++	Consuming any alcoholic beverage is associated with a decreased risk.
Reduced risk of forming gallstones	++	++	++	Consuming any alcoholic beverage is associated with a decreased risk.
Protection from the common cold		+		Only wine drinking is associated with protection from the common cold.

Better bone health	++	+	+	Silicon, which is present in beer but not in wine or liquor, has a beneficial effect on bone health.
Protection from age-related dementia/Alzheimer's disease	+	++	+	Alcohol has protective effects against dementia and Alzheimer's disease but wine may be superior to beer or liquor in the elderly population. Resveratrol found in abundance in grape skin and red wine has protective effects.
Increased longevity	++	+	+	Wine may provide the best effect.
Perception of good health		++		Only drinking wine is associated with subjective perception of good health.

++ Significant effect, + Positive effect

In general, there is a perception that red wine is superior to any other alcoholic beverages for providing many health benefits. Overall, consumers of alcoholic beverages perceive red wine to have more health benefits than beer and white wine (1). This perception may be partly due to the publication of a paper on French Paradox, showing the cardioprotective effects of wine.

French Paradox

French Paradox was first described by Professor Serge Renaud in a paper published in the prestigious medical journal, *Lancet*. In most countries, the high intake of saturated fat (eating food rich in fat) increases mortality from cardiovascular diseases, but the situation in France is paradoxical because mortality from cardiovascular diseases is relatively low compared to other industrialized countries such as the United Kingdom and the United States., despite the fact that French people consume fatty food. Professor Renaud attributed this paradox to their regular consumption of wine (20-30 gm per day: approximately 1 1/2 to2 glasses) In general, the moderate consumption of alcohol is associated with the reduced risk of cardiovascular diseases in the French population who mostly consume wine, the reduction of risk is more significant than consuming alcohol alone. This may be due to the presence of beneficial organic compounds in wine which can inhibit platelet inhibition, thus making the blood thin and reducing the risk of the formation of blood clots (2). A heart attack is due to the formation of a blood clot in the coronary artery which is already narrow due to plaque buildup (atherosclerosis; plaque consists of fat, cholesterol, calcium, and other compounds found in the blood). The blood clot may partially or completely block blood flow to the heart causing a heart attack where heart cells (cardiac myocytes) start dying due to the lack of oxygen.

Some researchers commented that red wine provides superior protection from cardiovascular diseases than any other alcoholic beverages due to the presence of resveratrol, a polyphenol. Red wine polyphenols are a complex mixture of various compounds which can be further classified as flavonoids (e.g., anthocyanins and flavan-3-ols) and non-flavonoids (e.g., resveratrol, cinnamates, and gallic acid). Although beneficial polyphenols such as catechin, para-coumaric acid, quercetin, kaempferol, hesperidin, gallic acid, and caffeic acid are found in wine, these beneficial compounds are also present in some fruits, vegetables, tea, and coffee. Resveratrol, a non-flavonoid polyphenol, is found exclusively in the skin of grapes and as a result this compound is found in a higher concentration in red wine than in white wine. However, not all red wines contain comparable amounts of resveratrol because depending on the geographical areas of the production of wine, the kind of vine, and the manufacturing process, resveratrol may vary from 0.09 mg/L to 7 mg/L (3).

Can All Alcoholic Beverages Protect from Cardiovascular Diseases?

The mechanisms by which alcoholic beverages exert their protective effects against cardiovascular diseases involve lipid regulation and systematic anti-inflammatory effects. The alcohol component of alcoholic beverages is responsible for increasing high-density lipoprotein cholesterol (HDL-cholesterol, also called good cholesterol), and inhibiting platelet aggregation. Alcohol also reduces systematic inflammation thus reducing the risk of cardiovascular diseases. Some studies indicate that red wine may be superior to white wine, beer, or sprit for cardioprotection because resveratrol found in higher amounts in red wine is very effective in preventing LDL (low-density lipoprotein, also called bad cholesterol) oxidation. Oxidized LDL has a higher tendency of depositing on coronary arteries causing plaque formation. Moreover, the polyphenolic components of red wine can further inhibit platelets, reduce inflammation, and activate proteins that prevent cell death. The effects are weaker in the case of white wine or beer due to lower concentrations of polyphenols compared to red wine (4).

However, there are also published reports indicating that white wine also has cardioprotective effects. Samuel et al. commented that white wine is equally cardioprotective as red white because white wine contains phenolic compounds such as tyrosol which has cardioprotective properties (5). Xiang et al. (2014) observed that the contribution percentage of resveratrol to the antioxidant activity of red wine was less than other polyphenols present in red wine. The highest antioxidant capacity was exhibited by para-coumaric acid. In addition, the resveratrol concentration varied from 0.80 mg/L to 4.61 mg/L (6). Falchi et al. (2006) concluded that the flesh of grapes is equally cardioprotective as skin, and the antioxidant capacity of skin and flesh of grapes are comparable (7). This observation further explains why white wine also has cardioprotective effects.

Beer is also rich in phenols and polyphenols which are antioxidants. Various studies have also shown the cardioprotective effect of beer. Cleophas (1999) concluded that any alcoholic beverage (wine, beer, or spirits) is associated with a slightly reduced risk of mortality and cardiovascular diseases (8). In a consensus document, the authors commented that the moderate consumption of beer (up to 1 drink a day in women, and up to 1 drink a day for men) reduces the risk of cardiovascular diseases and the effect is similar to that of wine (9). Rimm and Stampfer (2002) commented that beer and wine may have similar cardioprotective effects although in one study, the authors observed a 32% risk reduction in wine drinkers, and a 22% risk reduction in beer drinkers, but other studies observed no difference between beer and wine drinkers. In another study, the authors observed a 25% risk reduction in wine drinkers and a 23% risk reduction in beer drinkers (10).

Increased concentration of homocysteine, a naturally occurring amino acid in blood, is associated with an increased risk of cardiovascular disease. Homocysteine concentration in the blood is increased in alcoholics making them more susceptible to cardiovascular diseases. Although the moderate consumption of wine and spirits may slightly increase the level of homocysteine in blood, drinking beer has no effect on blood homocysteine levels. In one study, the authors observed an 8% increase in homocysteine levels in subjects after consumption of red wine for three weeks. Consumption of spirit for the same amount of time was associated with a 9% increase in homocysteine (such increases may increase the risk of cardiovascular diseases by

10-20%) but no increase was observed in subjects consuming beer (11).

Chiva-Blanch et al. (2013) compared the effects of wine, spirits, and beer on the protection against cardiovascular diseases and concluded that wine and beer (but especially red wine) seem to confer greater cardiovascular protection than spirits because of their polyphenolic content (12). Based on a review of medical literature, this author thinks that drinking beer and wine may be more beneficial than drinking spirits for cardiac health. Between beer and wine, wine, especially red wine, may provide a little additional protection from cardiovascular diseases. In an interesting study, Barefoot et al. (2002) concluded that the apparent health benefits of wine compared to other alcoholic beverages as reported by other investigators, may be a result of cofounding by dietary habits and by other lifestyle factors. The authors observed that subjects who preferred wine had healthier diets than those who preferred beer or sprits or who had no preferences. Wine drinkers also reported eating more servings of fruits and vegetables and fewer servings of red or fried meat. In addition, wine drinkers were less likely to smoke (13). Smoking increases the risk of cardiovascular diseases. In another study, the authors, based on results of the Copenhagen Health City Survey (12,039 subjects) concluded that light to moderate wine intake is related to good self-perceived health whereas this is not the case for beer and spirits (14).

Beneficial Antioxidant Compounds in Beer and Wine

Only part of the health benefits of drinking beer and wine is attributable to alcohol but many of its health benefits are due to the presence of many beneficial organic compounds, many of which are excellent antioxidants.

More than 2,000 compounds have been identified in various beers including more than 50 polyphenolic compounds because barley and hops are rich in many organic compounds including antioxidant polyphenolic compounds. Beer is also rich in nutrients including carbohydrates, amino acids, minerals, and vitamins. Beer is a good source of dietary antioxidants because 1 L of beer contains 366-875 mg of polyphenolic compounds (15). Therefore, one bottle of beer (355 mL) contains approximately 130 to 311 mg of polyphenolic compound. Xanthohumol, a very potent antioxidant present in hop, is also present in beer. Human exposure to xanthohumol and related compounds such as isoxanthohumol are primarily through beer consumption. Studies have indicated that these compounds are broad spectrum anticancer agents. Moreover, kaempferol, quercetin, tyrosol, and ferulic acid are also present in beer. In addition, beer contains 8-prenylnargine, a phytoestrogen and other compounds which have estrogen-like activities. It may have beneficial effects in preventing hot flashes in menopausal women. However, women receiving hormone replacement therapy for menopausal symptoms should consult with their physicians regarding alcohol consumption because both wine and beer may increase estrogen levels in the blood, thus increasing the risk of breast cancer. Many of these beneficial polyphenolic antioxidants present in beers are well absorbed after beer consumption and can be detected in the blood thus significantly increasing its antioxidant activities. Usually, maximum antioxidant capacity in the blood is observed approximately one hour after beer consumption. In addition, wines are prepared from grapes which are rich in antioxidant polyphenolic compounds. After the harvest, the grapes are crushed and allowed to ferment. Red wine is made from the must (pulp) of red or black grapes together with the grape skins, while white wine is usually made by fermenting juice pressed from white grapes, but can also be made from must extracted from red grapes but containing very little or no grape skin. Grape skin is full of polyphenolic compounds and anthocyanins which are excellent antioxidants. Soleas et al. (1997) demonstrated that these compounds are found in more abundance in red wine compared to white wine (16). Jakubec et al. (2012) measured the total antioxidant capacity and total polyphenol content of various brands of red, rose, and white wines and observed the highest concentrations of polyphenolic compounds in red wine compared to other wines. Antioxidant activity was highest in red wine where 1 glass of red wine was equivalent to 2glasses of white wine or 2 cups of black tea (17).

Like beer, polyphenolic antioxidants are rapidly absorbed after the consumption of wine thus increasing the antioxidant capacity of the blood. Usually, the maximum antioxidant capacity of the blood is observed approximately 55 minutes after drinking wine. Resveratrol found in abundance in grape skin has been described as a strong antioxidant compound. In one study, the authors found approximately 73 micrograms of resveratrol in 1 oz of grape juice. In contrast, 1 oz of red wine contained an average 160 micrograms of resveratrol (18).

The antioxidant capacity of the blood is increased after drinking either beer or wine. Although the polyphenol content of red wine is higher than white wine or beer, using beta-carotene bleaching assays to estimate the antioxidant capacity of beer, white wine, and red wine, Di Pietro and Bamforth (2011) observed that beer showed a superior antioxidant capacity than red and white wine, although using other assays to estimate the antioxidant capacity, red wine outperformed beer and white wine. The authors commented that the superior performance of beer in the beta-carotene bleaching assay which assesses protection against lipid peroxidation, beer is superior to red and white wine in preventing the oxidation of lipids. The oxidation of lipid is associated with plaque formation in coronary arteries thus restricting blood flow to the heart (atherosclerosis). The authors further commented that any alcoholic beverages including white wine and beer when consumed in the same equivalent quantities on the basis of alcohol units, allows the same health benefits as red wine. Moreover, beer has substantially more nutritive value than wine due to the presence of vitamins and minerals (19).

Nutritional Value of Beer

In general, beer contains significantly more nutrients than wine. One can of beer usually contains 10-20 gm of carbohydrates (low carbohydrate beer: 2.5-10 gm) but wine has much less amounts of carbohydrates. However, very low amounts of sugar are also present in beer and wine. Beer also contains trace amounts of minerals such as calcium, iron, magnesium, phosphorus, potassium, sodium, zinc, copper, manganese, and selenium. Beer contains approximately 300 micrograms of fluoride accounting for 10% of the recommended dietary allowance for fluoride. Beer is also a rich source of silicon which is essential for the growth and development of bone and connective tissues. Although low in some vitamin B complexes, beer is a good source of folate and choline (9). Choline is an essential nutrient. In addition, more calories can be derived from drinking beer than wine or spirits.

A can of beer usually contains approximately 1gm of protein but no protein is usually present in wine. Moreover, the amount of carbohydrates is much lower in wine explaining lower calorie content. Although minerals such as calcium, magnesium, potassium, and iron are present in wine, no silicon is present in wine. However, manganese is present in good amounts in wine while manganese is present in trace amounts in beer. Both beer and wine contain beneficial antioxidants. Although polyphenols, which are antioxidants, are found in much higher amounts in wine than beer, antioxidants present in beer are more readily absorbed than the antioxidants present in wine. As a result, the antioxidant capacity of the blood after drinking beer is comparable to drinking wine. The nutritional comparison of beer and wine is listed in table 2.

Table 2. Comparison of beer and wine for nutritional values

Nutritional factor	Beer (per serving)	Wine (per serving)
Calories	153	Red wine: 125 White wine: 121
Carbohydrate	10-20 gm	2 gm in red wine, 1 gm in white wine
Cholesterol	0 mg	0 mg
Vitamin B complex	Small amount but folate content is high	Small amounts
Choline	70 mg	10 mg
Minerals	Small amounts of minerals	Small amounts of minerals but rich in manganese
Silicon	Good source of silicon	Trace amount
Antioxidant effect	Although wine has more antioxidant compounds than beer, antioxidants in beer are more readily absorbed providing comparable antioxidant defense in the blood	Comparable antioxidant effect in the blood after consuming beer or wine
Dietary fiber	Contains beneficial soluble dietary fiber	No dietary fiber
Potent compounds	Xanthohumol, 8-prenylnaringenin, flavones, proanthocyanidins, and many others	Resveratrol (red wine), tyrosol (white wine), anthocyanins, flavonols, catechins, and many others

Beer, Wine, and Spirits for Cancer Protection

Currently, the most convincing evidence of the health benefits of the moderate consumption of alcohol is the reduced risk of cardiovascular diseases. Moderate alcohol consumption may reduce risks of certain types of cancer but a number of studies reported in medical literature is much less than the number of studies published on the beneficial effect of the moderate consumption of alcohol on cardiac health. Moreover, there are also conflicting reports. Nevertheless, the consumption of wine may reduce the risk of colon, basal cell carcinoma, ovarian, prostate, and renal cell carcinoma. Wine may also reduce the risk of lung cancer even in smokers (smoking is a risk factor for lung cancer). Compared to nondrinkers, women who consumed alcohol for at least 25 years previously were 33% less likely to die from cancer and 26% less likely to experience a relapse. Resveratrol, a component of red wine, has anticancer effects.

Xanthohumol, a component of hop which is also found in beer, is a potent anticancer agent. Other anticancer agents found in beer include 8-prenilnaringen, flavones, and proanthocyanidins. Beer drinking is associated with a significant reduction in prostate cancer in men compared to nondrinkers. However, alcohol use is related to cancer, most commonly cancer of the oral cavity. Even consuming more than 2 drinks a day for men, and more than 1 drink a day for women on a regular basis, increases the risk of cancer. The relation between alcohol consumption and breast cancer in women is controversial but consuming less than 3alcoholic beverages per week by women should not significantly increase the risk of breast cancer (see chapter 3). In general, beneficial antioxidants and anticancer agents present in beer and wine are responsible for protection because alcohol itself has no anticancer effect. In fact alcohol may act as a carcinogen (cancer-producing compound) for breast cancer.

Beer, Wine, Sprits, and Other Health Benefits of Moderate Alcohol Consumption

The moderate consumption of beer, wine, or spirits may reduce the risk of ischemic stroke but drinking more than 2drinks a day increases the risk of hemorrhagic stroke. Similarly, any type of alcoholic beverage may reduce the risk of type 2 diabetes. Drinking all types of alcohol (beer, wine, and liquor) was associated with the reduced risk of rheumatoid arthritis (see chapter 3). The moderate consumption of alcoholic beverages is beneficial for bones in men and in postmenopausal women. Silicone present in beer but not in wine or liquor has beneficial effects on bone health (20).

Drinking in moderation is associated with increased longevity. Poikolainen (1995) commented that the lowest risk of death seems to be at the average intake of 1 drink per day. However, there is no major difference between beer, wine, or liquor (21). In another cohort study, the authors concluded that low frequent use of any alcoholic beverage was associated with lower all-cause mortality as well as with mortality from cardiovascular diseases (22). However, based on a study of 13,064 men and 11, 459 women, Gronbaek et al. (1999) observed that compared to nondrinkers, light drinkers who avoided wine had a 10% lower chance of mortality but wine drinkers had a 34% lower chance of mortality (23). In another study, the authors concluded that light drinkers of any kind of wine had lower mortality risks than beer or liquor drinkers (24).

Beer Wine, Sprits, and Protection from Dementia/ Alzheimer's Disease

In general, moderate drinking is associated with a reduced risk of dementia and Alzheimer's disease, but heavy consumption alcohol increases the risk of dementia and cognitive impairment. Some studies observed no difference between alcoholic beverages in providing protection from age-related dementia and Alzheimer's disease, but other studies have indicated the superiority of wine (25). Studies have shown that for people 65 years of age and older who live in the Bordeaux region of France, moderate consumption of wine was associated with a lower risk of Alzheimer's disease and dementia. However, both the Canadian Study of Health and Aging and the Copenhagen

City Study involving subjects 55 years of age and older observed that light to moderate drinking was associated with a 42% reduction in the development of any dementia compared to nondrinkers regardless of drinking wine, beer, or liquor. Moreover, in the Nurses Health Study involving 12,000 retired nurses ages 70-81, moderate drinking was associated with a 20% less risk of cognitive impairment compared to nondrinkers. In this study, all types of alcoholic beverages had the same effect (26).

Kok et al. (2016) reported that like wine, beer drinking also protects against Aβ-aggregation of β-amyloid peptide in the brain, the triggering agent for Alzheimer's disease (27). However, other studies have shown that wine is superior in providing protection against Alzheimer's disease. Braidy et al. (2016) commented that apart from being an antioxidant, resveratrol is effective in protecting the brain from the development of the neurotoxic Aβ-aggregation of β-amyloid peptide in the brain as well as having the ability to remove such aggregates. Resveratrol can break down the precursor of protein that is associated with Aβ-aggregation. The authors further commented that resveratrol is a potential therapeutic candidate for the treatment of Alzheimer's disease (28).

Unique Health Benefits of Beer

Only beer contains soluble dietary fibers. These are beta-linked compounds derived from the betaglycan and arabinoxylane present in barley. Such materials are neither modified by brewer yeast nor metabolized by the human body. As a result, these compounds, known as dietary fibers, pass through the body to the large intestine. Soluble dietary fibers have many health benefits including binding cholesterol (that has a positive effect on the health of the heart) and healthy bowel movements; these substances also have positive effects on the beneficial bacteria of the lower gut. Beer may contain 2 gm/L of dietary fiber but some may contain two to threefold more dietary fiber (29).

Only beer is a rich source of folate and drinking beer is associated with good blood levels of folate and vitamin B12 which lower the homocysteine concentration in the blood. Higher blood levels of homocysteine are associated with an increased risk of cardiovascular diseases. Mayer (2001) concluded that moderate beer consumption may help to maintain the homocysteine level within the normal range in the blood due to its high folate content (30). This is a unique feature of beer because wine and spirits may slightly increase the blood homocysteine level.

Beer is slightly more effective in lowering the risk of kidney stones than other alcoholic beverages. In one study based on 194,095 participants, the authors concluded that consumption of sugar-sweetened sodas and punch was associated with a higher risk of kidney stone formation, whereas the moderate consumption of beer was associated with a 41% lower risk. Consuming wine was associated with a 31-33% lower risk while orange juice reduced the risk by 12%. Drinking caffeinated coffee may lower the risk by 26%, while decaffeinated coffee may lower the risk by 16% and tea may lower the risk by 11% (31).

Moderate beer consumption has beneficial effects on the immune system but such effects are more significant in women (32). Although there is a popular belief that beer is good pre-exercise hydration beverage, in reality, only drinking nonalcoholic beer is beneficial as pre-exercise drink. Drinking alcoholic beer may negatively affect health and physical performance during exercise by lowering the sodium level and by increasing the potassium level in plasma (aqueous portion of blood) (33). There is a popular belief that consuming beer may cause weight gain due to its higher calorie content compared to wine. However, epidemiological studies clearly indicate that the moderate consumption of beer is not associated with weight gain. However, the heavy consumption of any alcoholic beverage (30 gm or more alcohol per day, more than 2 drinks a day) is associated with weight gain.

Unique Health Benefits of Wine

Some of the health benefits of wine may be related to different demographics of people who prefer wine versus beer. As mentioned earlier in the chapter, wine drinkers usually have healthier diets than beer drinkers. Moreover, wine drinkers have a much lower prevalence of smoking than beer drinkers. In one study involving 12, 958 young adults, the authors observed that wine drinkers generally had more formal education, better dietary and exercise habits, and more favorable health status indicators such as normal body mass index than beer or spirit drinkers. In addition, a large portion of wine drinkers were light to moderate drinkers compared to beer or liquor drinkers. In addition, wine drinkers were less likely to report smoking or problems drinking than beer or liquor drinkers (34).

Sluik et al. (2016) reported that wine consumers had higher levels of good cholesterol (HDL-cholesterol), lower hemoglobin A1C (lower levels indicate better sugar control over the last 120 days), and were more likely to follow the salad pattern of diet (high intake of vegetables, fish, fruits, soup, and eggs, low intake of sweets, snacks, cake, and cookies). In contrast, beer consumers had the highest levels of triglycerides and liver enzymes and also consumed more meat and bread. The authors concluded that wine drinkers had overall better health than beer or spirit drinkers (35). In another study involving a 29-year follow-up of mortality and quality of life, the authors observed that wine was associated with a lower mortality and quality of life in old age (36). Moderate wine drinking reduced the risk of hip fractures in postmenopausal women compared to beer drinkers and hard liquor drinkers (37). Xu et al. (2015), based on a review of eight publications and meta-analyses, concluded that wine consumption among females reduced the risk of renal cell carcinoma (the most common type of kidney cancer). However, in males only beer drinking was associated with a reduced risk of this type of cancer (38). Light to moderate consumption of wine may protect against weight gain (39).

Beer, Wine, or Vodka: What Should I Drink?

Overall, the alcohol content of alcoholic beverages is associated with many health benefits of drinking in moderation. The practice of drinking in moderation (up to 1drink a day for women, and up to 2drinks a day for men) is more important than the selection of beverage type. Drinking in excess regardless of beverage type is harmful. Interestingly, social and occasional drinkers also get health benefits of alcohol consumption. Women even consuming 1 drink per week or less get protection from cardiovascular diseases, but men need to drink a little more frequently to get the full benefits of light drinking. Interestingly, the health benefits of light to moderate drinking is more significant in older men than in younger men but women of any age may get these health benefits.

For drinking preferences, beer and wine almost have almost similar beneficial effects. Red wine may have slightly more beneficial effects than beer or white wine, but contrary to popular belief, red wine is not a miracle drink because drinking white wine and beer has many health benefits too. Drinking beer and white wine may provide similar antioxidant defenses of the blood. However, for the older population (65 years or older), red wine appears to have more benefits than white wine or beer. However, for women of any age, wine (both red and white) appears to be little more beneficial than beer.

Both beer and wine have carbohydrates and other nutrients but liquors (distilled alcoholic drinks, e.g., vodka, rum, or whiskey) do not contain any carbohydrates or significant amounts of vitamins. However, during aging using wood barrels, beneficial polyphenols may leak into distilled spirits. Aging of wine using oak barrels also enriches wine with polyphenols present in oak wood. However, it is advisable to drink wine and beer more often. If you like to drink liquor, consider drinking a cocktail because fruit juices are rich sources of polyphenolic antioxidants and vitamins, especially vitamin C.

Overall, men prefer drinking beer and women prefer wine. For men below 50 years of age, drinking beer in moderation is fine. However, for older men, especially men over 65 years of age, drinking wine, especially red wine, has more benefits including a significant reduction of risk of dementia and Alzheimer's disease. Moreover, wine consumption in the elderly population is associated with an overall perception of good health but drinking beer or sprit does not provide that benefit. Therefore, drinking more wine than beer or spirits may be beneficial for elderly people.

For women who prefer drinking wine, continue your choice. Both white and red wine have health benefits. If you prefer to drink beer, consider drinking wine, especially red wine occasionally. For elderly women, drinking wine has more benefits. Therefore, consider drinking wine more often than beer or cocktails.

Conclusions

Drinking in moderation is the key to good health and beverage preference is less important. However, this author recommends consuming beer or wine more frequently than liquors. If your preference is pina colada or another cocktail, that is fine too but also try to drink beer or wine more frequently because all fruit drinks containing alcohol are high in calories. For younger men, if you prefer beer, continue to drink in moderation but when you get older; consider drinking wine, especially red wine more frequently than drinking beer. In general, women get slightly more benefits from drinking wine and if you love beer, consider drinking wine sometimes. The relationship between alcohol consumption and the risk of breast cancer is controversial. If you have a family history of breast cancer, consult your physician regarding alcohol consumption. Also, consult with your physician if you are receiving hormone replacement therapy for menopause. Even the moderate consumption of alcohol (2 drinks a day for men) may negatively impact a patient with HIV infection. Again, talk to your physician.

BIBLIOGRAPHY

Chapter 1
1. Erol A. & Karpyak, V. M. Sex and gender related differences in alcohol use and its consequences: Contemporary knowledge and future research considerations. Drug Alcohol Depend 2015; 156: 1-13.
2. Lotfipour S., Cisneros, V., Ogbu, U. C., McCoy, C. E., et al. A retrospective analysis of ethnic and gender differences in alcohol consumption among emergency department patients: A cross-sectional study. BMC Emerg Med 2015; 29: 24.
3. Dudley, R. Ethanol, fruit ripening and the historical origins of human alcoholism in primate frugivory. Integra Comp Biol 2004; 44 (4): 315-323.
4. Vallee, B. L. Alcohol in the Western world. Scientific American 1998; 278 (6): 80-85.
5. Loyola Marymount University, Los Angeles heads up: History of alcohol use http://academics.lmu.edu/headsup/forstudents/historyofalcoholuse. Accessed June 11, 2016.
6. Jones, J. M. US drinkers divide between beer and wine as favorite. Gallup poll

http:www.galluppoll/poll/163787/drinkers-
divide-beer-wine-favorite.aspx
Accessed June 19, 2016.

7. Lieber, C. S. The influence of alcohol on nutritional
    status. Nutr Rev 1988; 46: 241-254.

8. Hoyumpa, A. M. Mechanism of vitamin
    deficiencies in alcoholics. Alcohol Clin Exp Res
    1986; 10: 573-581.

9. Gloria, L., Cravo, M., Camilo, M. E., Resende, M.,
    et al. Nutritional deficiencies in chronic alcoholics:
    Relation to dietary and alcohol consumption. Am J
    Gasteroenterol 1997; 92: 485-489.

Chapter 2

1. Celik, S., Karapirli, M., Kandemir, E., Ucar, F., Kantarci, M. N., Gurler, M. *et al.* Fatal ethyl and methyl alcohol related poisoning in Ankara: Aretrospective analysis of 10,720 cases between 2001 and 2011. J Forensic Leg Med 2013; 20: 151-154.

2. Lac, A., & Donaldson, C. D. Alcohol attitudes, motives, norms and personality traits longitudinally classify nondrinkers, moderate drinkers and binge drinkers using discriminant function analysis. Addict Behav 2016; 61: 91-98.

3. Marczinski, C. A. Can energy drinks increase the desire for more alcohol? Ad Nutr 2015; 6: 96-101.

4. McCartt, A. T., Hellinga, L. A., & Kirley, B. B. The effect of minimum legal drinking age 21 laws on alcohol related driving in the United States. J Safety Res 2010; 41: 173-181.

5. Carpenter, C., & Dobkin, C. The minimum legal drinking age and public health. J Econ Perspect 2011; 25: 133-156.

6. Silveri, M. M. Adolescent brain development and underage drinking in the United States: Identifying risks of alcohol use in college populations. Harv Rev Psychiatry 2012; 20: 189-200.

7. Jones, A. W., & Jonsson, K. A. Food-induced lowering of blood ethanol profiles and increased rate of elimination immediately after a meal. J Forensic Sci 1994; 39: 1084-1093.

8. Jones, A. W. Evidence based survey of the literature of the elimination rates of ethanol from blood with applications in forensic casework.

Forensic Sci Int 2010; 200: 1-20.

9. Marshall, A. W., Kingstone, D., Boss, M., & Morgan, M. Y. Ethanol elimination in males and females: Relationship to menstrual cycle and body composition. Hepatology 1983; 3: 701-706.

10. Gill, J. Women alcohol and the menstrual cycle. Alcohol and Alcoholism (April 1997); 32 (4): 435-441.

11. Dufour, M. C., Archer L., & Gordis, E. Alcohol and elderly. Clin Geriatr Med 1992; 8: 127-141.

12. Caputo, C., Wood, E., & Jabbour, L. Impact of fetal alcohol exposure on body system: A systematic review. Birth Defect Res C Embryo Today 2016; 108: 174-180.

13. Haastrup, M. B., Pottegard, A., & Damkier. P. Alcohol and breastfeeding. Basic Clin Pharamcol Toxicol 2014; 114: 168-173.

14. Falleti, M. G., Maruff, P., Collie, A., Darby, D. G. et al. Qualitative similarities in cognitive impairment associated with 24 g of sustained wakefulness and blood alcohol concentration of 0.05%. J Sleep Res 2003; 12: 265-274.

15. Fell, J. C., &Voss, R. B. The effectiveness of a 0.05% blood alcohol concentration (BAC) limit for driving in the United States. Addiction 2014; 109: 869-874.

16. Hlastala, M. P., & Anderson, J. C. The impact of breathing pattern and lung size on the alcohol breath test. Ann Biomed Eng 2007; 35: 264-272.

Chapter 3

1. Numminen, H., Syrjala, M., Benthin, G., Kaste, M. et al. The effects of acute ingestion of a large dose of alcohol on the hemostatic system and its circadian variation. Stroke 2000; 31: 1269-1273.

2. Garcia-Moreno, H., Calvo, J. R., & Maldonado, M. D. High levels of melatonin generated during the brewing process. J Pineal Res 2013; 55: 26-30.

3. Murch, S. J., Hall, B. A., Le, C. H., & Saxena, P. K. Changes in the levels of indoleamine phytochemicals during veraison and ripening of wine grapes. J Pineal Res 2010; 49: 95-100.

4. Friedman, L. A., & Kimball, A. W. Coronary heart disease mortality and alcohol consumption in Framingham. Am J Epidemiol 1986; 124: 481-489.

5. Tolstrup, J., Jensen, M. K., Tjonneland, A., Overvad, K., Mukamal. K. J., & Gronbaek, M. 2006. Prospective study of alcohol drinking patterns and coronary heart disease in women and men. British Med J 2006; 332: 1244-1248.

6. O'Keefe, J. H., Bhatti, S. K., Bajwa, A., DiNicolantonio, J. et al. Alcohol and cardiovascular health: The dose makes the poison or the remedy. Mayo Clinic Proc 2014; 89: 382-293.

7. Gemes, K., Janszky, I., Laugsand, L. E., Laszlo, K. D. et al. Alcohol consumption is associated with a lower incident of acute myocardial infarction: Results from a large prospective population based study in Norway. J Intern Med 2016; 279: 365-375.

8. Rosenbloom, J. I., Mukamal, K. J., Frost, L. E., & Mittleman, M. A. Alcohol consumption patterns, beverage type, and long term mortality among women survivors of acute myocardial infarction.

Am J Cardiol 2012; 109: 147-152.

9. Wu, J. M., & Hiieh, T. C. Resveratrol: A cardioprotective substance. Ann NY Acad Sci 2011; 1215: 16-21.

10. Truelsen, T., Gronbaek, M., Schnohr, P., & Boyen, G. Intake of beer, wine and spirits and risk of stroke: The Copenhagen city heart study. Stroke 1998; 29: 2467-2472.

11. Elkind, M., Sciacca, R., Boden-Albala, B., Rundek, T. et al. Moderate alcohol consumption reduces risk of ischemic stroke. The Northern Manhattan study. Stroke 2006; 37: 13-19.

12. Saco, R. L., Elkind, M., Boden-Albala, B., Lin, I. F. et al. The protective effect of moderate alcohol consumption on ischemic stroke. JAMA 1999; 281: 53-60.

13. Koppes, L. L, Dekker, J. M., Hendriks, H. F., Bouter, L. M., & Heine, R. J. Moderate alcohol consumption lowers the risk of Type 2 diabetes: A meta-analysis of prospective observational studies. Diabetes Care 2005; 28 (3): 719-725.

14. Pietraszek, A., Gregersen, S., & Hermansen, K. Alcohol and type 2 diabetes: A review. Nutr Metab Cardiovasc Dis 2010; 20: 366-375.

15. Chao, C., Slezak, J. M., Caan, B. J, & Quinn, V. P. Alcoholic beverage intake and risk of lung cancer: The California Men's Health Study. Cancer Epidemiol Biomarkers Prev 2008; 17: 2692-2699.

16. Pelucchi, C., Galeone, C., Montella, M., Polesel, J., Crispo, A., Talamini, R. et al. Alcohol consumption and renal cell cancer risk in two Italian case controlled study. Ann Oncology 2008; 19: 1003-1008.

17. Pelucchi, C., Tramacere, I., Boffetta, P., Negri, E. et al. Alcohol consumption and cancer risk. Nutr Canver 2011; 63: 983-980.

18. Lowry, S. J., Kappahahn, K., Chlebowski, R. T., &

Li, C. I. Alcohol use and breast cancer survival among participants in the women's health initiative. Cancer Epidemiol Biomarker Prev 2016; May 19 [e-pub ahead of print].

19. Strumylaite, L., Sharp, S. J., Kregzdyte, R., Poskiene, L. et al. The association of low to moderate alcohol consumption with breast cancer subtypes defined by hormone receptor status. PLoS One 2015; 10: e0144680.

20. Kallberg, H., Jacobsen, S., Bengtsson, C., Pedersen, M. et al. 2009. Alcohol consumption is associated with decreased risk of rheumatoid arthritis: Results from two Scandinavian studies. Ann Rheumatoid Dis 68: 222-227.

21. Nissen, M. J., Gabay, C., Scherer, A., & Finchk, A. 2010. The effect of alcohol on radiographic progression in rheumatoid arthritis. Arthritis Rheum 62: 1265-1272.

22. Di Giuseppe, D., Alfredsson, L., Bottai, M., Askling, J. et al. Long term alcohol intake and risk of arthritis in women: A population based cohort study. British Med J 2012; 345: e4230.

23. Leitzmann, M. F., Giovannucci, E. L., Stampfer, M. J., Spiegelman, D. et al. Prospective study of alcohol consumption patterns in relation to symptomatic gallstone disease in man. Alcohol Clin Exp Res 1999; 23: 835-841.

24. Takkouch, B., Regueira-Mendez, C., Garcia-Closas, R., Figueiras, A., Gestal-Oterro, J. J. & Hernan, M. A. Intake of wine, beer, and spirits and the risk of clinical common cold. Am J Epidemiol 2002; 155: 853-858.

25. Klatsky, A. L., Friedman, G. D., & Siegekaub, A. B. Alcohol and mortality: A ten year Kaiser-Permanente experience. Ann Int Med 1981; 95: 139-145.

26. Camargo, C. A., Hennekens, C. H., Gaziano, J. M.,

Glynn, R. J. et al. Prospective study of moderate alcohol consumption and mortality in US male physicians. Arch Int Med 1997: 157: 79-85.

27. Clarisse, R, Testu, F., & Reinberg, A. Effect of alcohol on psycho-technical test and social communication in a festive situation: a Chrono psychological approach. Chronobiolo Int 2004; 21: 721-738.

28. Peele, S., & Brodsky A. Exploring psychological benefits associated with moderate alcohol use: A necessary corrective to assessments of drinking outcomes? Drug Alcohol Depend 2000; 60: 221-247.

29. Gonzalez-Rubio, E., San Mauro, I., Lopez-Ruiz, C., Diaz-Prieto, L. E. et al. Relationship of moderate alcohol intake and type of beverage with health behaviors and quality of life in elderly. Qual Life Res 2016 Jan 21 [e-pub ahead of print].

30. Parodi, J., Ormeno, D., & Ochoa-de la Paz, L.D. Amyloid pore channel hypothesis: effect of ethanol on aggregation state using frog oocytes for an Alzheimer's disease study. BMB Rep 2015; 48: 13-18.

31. Pasinetti, G. M., Wang, J., Jo, L; Zhao, W. et al. Roles of resveratrol and other grape-derived polyphenols in Alzheimer's disease prevention and treatment. Biochem Biophys Acta 2015; 1852: 1202-1208.

Chapter 4
1. Roerecke, M., & Rehm, J. Irregular heavy drinking occasions and risk of ischemic cardiovascular disease: A systematic review and meta-analysis. Am J Epidemiol 2010; 171 (6): 633-644.
2. Miller, J. W., Naimi, T. S., Brewer, R. D., & Jones, S. E. Binge drinking and associated health risk behaviors among high school students. Pediatrics 2007; 19: 76-85.
3. Jennisom, K. M. The short term effects and unintended long term consequences of binge drinking in college: A 10 year follow-up study. Am J Drug Alcohol Abuse 2004; 30: 659-684.
4. Naimi, T. S., Brewer, R. D., Miller, J. W., Okoro, C. et al. What do binge drinkers drink? Implications for alcohol control policy. Am J Prev Med 2004; 33: 188-193.
5. Graff-Iversen, S., Jansen, M. D., Hoff, D. A., Hoiseth, G. et al. Divergent associations of drinking frequency and binge consumption of alcohol with mortality within same cohort. J Epidemiol Community Health 2013; 67: 350-357.
6. Kachele, M., Wolff, S., Kratzer, W., Haenle, M. et al. Presence of fatty liver and the relationship between alcohol consumption and markers of inflammation. Mediators Inflamm 2015; 2015:278785.
7. Belentani, S., & Tribelli, C. 2001. Spectrum of liver disease in general population. Lessons from Dionysus study. J Hepatol 2001; 35: 531-537.
8. Bellentani, S., Saccoccio, G., Costa, G., Tribelli, C., Manenti, F., Sodde, M. et al. Drinking habits as cofactors of risk of alcohol induced liver damage Gut 1997; 42: 845-850.
9. Walsh, K., & Alexander, G. Alcoholic liver disease.

Postgrad Med 2000; 281: 280-286.

10. Hezode, C., Lonjon, I., Roudot-Thorval, F., Pawlotsky, J. M. et al. Impact of moderate alcohol consumption on histological activity and fibrosis in patients with chronic hepatitis C, and specific influence of steatosis, a prospective study. Aliment Pharmacol Ther 2003; 17: 1031-1037.

11. Medina, K. L., McQueeny, T., Nagel, B. J., Hanson, K. L., Schweinsburg, A. D., & Tapert, S. E. Prefrontal cortex volumes in adolescents with alcohol use disorders: Unique gender effects. Alcohol Clin Exp Res 2008; 32: 386-394.

12. Kopelman, M. D., Thomson, A. D., Guerrini, I., & Marshall, E. J. 2009. The Korsakoff syndrome: Clinical aspect, psychology and treatment. Alcohol Alcoholism 44: 148-154.

13. Harper, C. 2007. The neurotoxicity of alcohol. Hum Exp Toxicol 2007; 26: 251-257.

14. Trabert, W., Betz, T., Niewald, M., & Huber, G. Significant reversibility of alcohol brain shrinkage within 3 weeks of abstinence. Acta Psychia Scand 1995; 92: 87-90.

15. Laonigro, I., Correale, M., Di Biase, M., & Altomare, E. 2009. Alcohol abuse and heart failure. Eu J Heart Failure 11: 453-462.

16. Yedlapati, S. H., Mendu, A., & Stewart, S. H. Alcohol related diagnoses and increased mortality in acute myocardial infarction patients: An analysis of nationwide inpatient sample. J Hosp Med 2016; April 4 [e-pub ahead of print].

17. Ikehara, S., Iso, H., Yamagishi, K., & Yamamoto, S. 2009. Alcohol consumption, social support and risk of stroke and coronary cardiovascular disease among Japanese men: The JPHC study. Alcohol Clin Exp Res 33: 1025-1032.

18. Martin-Moreno, J. M., Boyle, P., Gorgojo, L., Willett, W. C., Gonzalez, J., Villar, F. et al. 1993.

Alcoholic beverage consumption and risk of breast cancer in Spain. Cancer Causes Control 1993; 4: 345-353.

19. Bessaoud, F., & Daures, J. P. 2008. Pattern of alcohol (especially wine) consumption and breast cancer risk: A case controlled study among population in Southern France. Ann Epidemiol 18: 467-475.

20. Nagata, C., Mizoue, T., Tanaka, K., Tsuji, I., Wakai, K., Inoue, M. et al. 2007. Alcohol drinking and breast cancer risk: An evaluation based on a systematic review of epidemiological evidence among Japanese population. Jpn J Clin Oncol 2007; 37; 568-574.

21. Pelucchi, C., Tramacere, I., Boffetta, P., Negri, E. et al. Alcohol consumption and cancer risk. Nutr Canver 2011; 63: 983-980.

22. Baum, M. K., Rafie, C., Lai, C., Sales, S., Page, J. B., & Campa, A. Alcohol use accelerates HIV disease progression. AIDS Res Hum Retrovir. 2010; 26: 511-518.

23. Guthauser, B., Boitrelle, F., Plat, A., Thiercelin, N. et al. Chronic excessive alcohol consumption and male fertility: A case report on reversible azoospermia and a literature review. Alcohol Alcoholism 2014; 49: 42-44.

24. Emanuele, N., & Emanuele, M. A. Alcohol alters critical hormonal balance. Alcohol Health Res World 1997; 21: 53-64.

25. May, P. A., & Gossage, J. P. Estimating the prevalence of fetal alcohol syndrome: A summary. Alcohol Res Health 2001; 25: 159-167.

26. Blow F. C., Brockmann, L. M., & Barry, K. L. Role of alcohol in late-life suicide. Alcohol Clin Exp Res 2004; 28: 5 Supply: 48 S-56S.

27. Palijan, T. Z., Kovacevic, D., Radeljak, S., Kovac, M., & Mustapic, J. Forensic aspects of alcohol

abuse and homicide. Coll Antropol 2009; 33: 893-897.

28. Quigley, B. M., & Leonard, K. E. Alcohol and the continuation of early marital aggression. Alcohol Clin Exp Res 2000; 24: 1003-1010.

29. Dawson, D. A. Alcohol and mortality from external causes. J Stu Alcohol Drug. 2001; 62(6): 790-797.

30. Hart, C. L., Smith, G. D., Hole, D.J., & Hawthorne, V. M. Alcohol consumption and mortality from all causes, coronary cardiovascular disease, and stroke: Results from a prospective cohort study of Scottish men with 21 years of follow up. BMJ 1999; 318 (7200): 1725-1729.

31. Britton, A., & Marmot, M. Different measures of alcohol consumption and risk of coronary cardiovascular disease and all-cause mortality: An11 year follow up of the Whitehall II cohort study. Addiction 2004; 99: 109-116.

32. Anda, R. F., Williamson, D. F., & Remington, P. L. Alcohol and fatal injuries among US adults. Finding from the NHANES I Epidemiologic follow up study. JAMA 1998; 260 (17): 2529-2532.

33. Schilling, E. A., Aseltine, R. H., Glanovsky, J. L., James, A., & Jacobs, D. Adolescent alcohol use, suicidal indention and suicide attempts. J Adolesc Health 2009; 44: 335-341.

34. Kanny, D., Brewer, R. D., Mesnick, J. B., Paulozzi, L. J. et al. MMWR Morb Mortal Wkly Rep 2015 63: 1238-1242.

Chapter 5

1. Tomcikova, Z., Veselska, Z.D., Geckova, A.M. van Dijk, J.P. et al. Adolescents drinking and drunkenness more likely in one parent families and due to poor communication with mother. Cent Eur J Public Health 2015; 23: 54-58.

2. Van der Vorst, H., Engles, R. C., Meeus, W., & Dekovic, M. The impact of alcohol-specific rules, parental norms about early drinking and parental alcohol use on adolescent's drinking behavior. J Child Psychol Psychiatry 2006; 47: 1299-1306.

3. Skinner, M. L., Hong, S., Herrenkohl, T. I., & Brown, E. C. Longitudinal effects of early childhood maltreatment on the co-occurring substance misuse and mental health problems in adulthood: The role of adolescent alcohol use and depression. J Stud Alcohol Drugs 2016; 77: 464-472.

4. Smith, C. A., Elwyn, L. K., Ireland, T. O., & Thornberry, T. P. Impact of adolescent exposure to intimate partner violence on substance use in early adulthood. J Stud Alcohol Drugs 2010; 71: 219-230.

5. Keyes, K. M., Hatzenbuehler, M. L., Grant, B. F., & Hasin, D. S. Stress and alcohol: epidemiological evidence. Alcohol Res Curr Review 2012; 34: 391-400

6. Kendler, K. S., Lonn, S. L., Salvatore, J., Sundquist, J. et al. Effect of marriage on risk of onset of alcohol use disorder: A longitudinal and co-relative analysis in a Swedish national sample. Am J Psychiatry 2016; May 16 [e-pub ahead of print].

7. Reddy, S., Dick, A. M., Geber, M. R., & Mitchell, K. The effect of a yoga intervention on alcohol and

drug abuse risk in veteran and civilian women in posttraumatic stress syndrome. J Altern Complement Med 2014; 20: 75-756.

8. McCree, R. R., & John, O. P. An introduction to five factor model and its applications. J Pers 1992; 60: 175-215.

9. Martin, E. D., Sher, K. J. Family history of alcoholism, alcohol use disorders and five factor model of personality. J Stud Alcohol 1994; 55: 81-90.

10. Bozkurt, M., Evren, C., Cay, Y., Evren, B. et al. Relationship of personality dimension with impulsivity in alcohol dependent inpatients men. Nord J Psychiatry 2014; 68: 316-322.

11. Kimura, M., & Higuchi, S. Genetics of alcohol dependence. Psychiatry Clin Neurosci 2011; 65: 213-225.

12. Lai, C. L., Yao, C.T., Chau, G. Y., Yang, L. F., Kuo, T.Y., Chiang, C.P. et al. Dominance of the inactive Asian variant over activity and protein contents of mitochondrial aldehyde dehydrogenase 2 in human liver. Alcohol Clin Exp Res 2014; 38: 44-50.

13. Wall, T. L., Shea, S. H., Luczak, S. E., Cook, T. A., & Carr, L. G. Genetic association of alcohol dehydrogenase with alcohol use disorders and endo phenotypes in white college students. J Abnorm Psychol 2005; 114: 456-465.

14. Carr, L. G., Foroud, T., Stewart, T., Castelluccio, P., Edenberg, H. J., & Li, T. K. Influence of ADH1B polymorphism on alcohol use and its subjective effects in Jewish population. Am J Med Genet 2002; 112: 138-143.

Chapter 6

1. Wright, C. A., Bruhn, C. M., Heymann, H., & Bamforth. C.W. Beer and wine consumer's perceptions of the nutritional value of alcoholic and nonalcoholic beverages. J Food Sci 2008; 73: H8-H11.

2. Renaud, S., & De Lorgeril, M. Wine, alcohol, platelet, and French paradox for coronary heart disease. Lancet 1992; 339: 1523-1526.

3. Biagi, M., & Bertelli, A. Wine alcohol and pills: What future for the French paradox? Life Sciences 2015; 131: 19-22.

4. Wu, J. M., Wang, Z. R., Hsieh, T. C., Bruder, J. L. et al. Mechanism of cardioprotection by resveratrol, a phenolic antioxidant present in red wine (review). Int J Mol Med 2001; 8: 3-17.

5. Samuel SM, Thirunavukkarasu M, Penumathsa SV, Paul D et al. Akt/FOXO3/SIRT1-mediated cardioprotection by n-tyrosol against ischemic stress in vivo model of myocardial infarction: Switching gears towards survival and longevity. J Argi Food Chem 2008; 56: 9692-9698.

6. Xiang, L., Xiao, L., Wang, Y., Li, H. et al. Health benefits of wine: Don't expect resveratrol too much. Food Chem 2014; 156: 258-263.

7. Falchi, M., Bertelli, A., Lo Scalzo, R., Morassut, M. et al. Comparison of cardioprotective abilities between flesh and skin of grapes. J Agri Food Chem 2006; 54: 6613-6622.

8. Cleophas, T. J. Wine, beer and spirits and risk of myocardial infarction: A systematic review. Biomed Pharamcother 1999; 53: 417-423.

9. De Gaetano, G., Costanzo, S., Di Castelnuvo, A., Badimon, L. et al. Effects of moderate beer consumption on health and disease: A consensus report. Nutr Metab Cardiovasc Dis 2016; 26: 443-

467.

10. Rimm, E. B., & Stampfer, M. J. Wine, beer and spirits: Are they really horses of a different color? Circulation 2002; 15: 2806-2807.

11. Van der Gaag, M. S., Ubbink, J. B., Sillanaukee, P., Nikkari, S. et al. Effect of consumption of red wine, spirits and beer on serum homocysteine. Lancet 2000; 255: 1522.

12. Chiva-Blanch, G., Arranz, S., Lamuela-Raventos, R. M., & Estruch, R. Effects of wine, alcohol and polyphenols on cardiovascular disease risk factors: Evidences from human studies. Alcohol Alcoholism 2013; 48: 270-277.

13. Barefoot, J. C., Gronbaek, M., Feaganes, J. R., McPherson, R. S. et al. Alcoholic beverage preference, diet, and health habits in UNC Alumni Heart Study. Am J Clin Nutr 2002; 76: 466-472.

14. Gronbaek, M., Mortensen, E. L., Mygind, K., Andersen, A. T. et al. Beer, wine, spirits and subjective health. J Epidemiol Community Health 1999: 53: 721-724.

15. Piazzon, A., Forte, M., & Nardini, M. Characterization of phenolic content and antioxidant activity of different beer types. J Agri Food Chem 2010; 58: 327-334.

16. Soleas, G. J., Diamandis, E. P., & Goldberg, D. M. Wine as a biological fluid: History, production and role in disease prevention. Journal of Clinical Laboratory Analysis.1997; 11: 287-313.

17. Jakubec P., Bancirova, M., Halouzka, V, Lojek, A. et al. Electrochemical sensing of total antioxidant capacity and polyphenol content in wine samples using amperometry online coupled with microdialysis. J Agri Food Chem 2012; 60: 7836-7843.

18. Brouillard, R., George, F., & Fougerousse, A. Polyphenols produced during red wine aging.

Biofactors 1997: 6: 403-410.

19. Di Pietro, M. B., & Bamforth, C.W. A comparison of the antioxidant potential of wine and beer. J Inst Brew 2011; 117: 547-555.

20. Tucker, K. L., Jugdaohsingh, R., Powell, J. J., Qiao, N. et al. Effects of beer, wine, and liquor intake on bone mineral density in older men and women. Am J Clin Nutr 2009; 89: 1188-1196.

21. Poikolainen, K. Alcohol and mortality: A review. J Clin Epidemiol 1995; 48: 455-465.

22. Graff-Iversen, S., Jansen, M. D., Hoff, D. A., Hoiseth, G. et al. Divergent associations of drinking frequency and binge consumption of alcohol with mortality within same cohort. J Epidemiol Community Health 2013; 67: 350-357.

23. Gronbaek, M., Becker, U., Johansen, D., Gottschau, A. et al. Type of alcohol consumed and mortality from all causes, coronary heart disease and cancer. Ann Intern Med 2000; 133: 411-419.

24. Klatsky, A. L., Friedman, C. D., Armstrong, M. A., & Kipp, H. Wine, liquor, beer and mortality. Am J Epidemiol 2003; 158: 585-595.

25. Neafsey, E. J., & Collins, M. A. Moderate alcohol consumption and cognitive risk. Neuropsychiatr Dis Treat 2011; 7: 465-484.

26. Sherman, F. T. The case for alcohol in the primary prevention of dementia: Abstinence may be bad for your health. Geriatrics 2006; 61: 10-12.

27. Kok, E. H., Karppinen, T. T., Luoto, T., Alafuzoff, I. et al. Beer drinking associates with lower burden of amyloid beta aggregation in the brain: Helsinki Sudden Death Series. Alcohol Clin Exp Res 2016; 40:1473-1478.

28. Braidy, N., Jugder, B. E., Poljak, A., Jayasena, T. et al. Resveratrol as a potential therapeutic candidate for the treatment and management of Alzheimer's disease. Curr Top Med Chem 2016; 16: 1951-1960.

29. Bamforth, C. W. Beer carbohydrate and diet. J Inst Brew 2005; 111: 259-264

30. Mayer, O. Jr, Simon, J., & Rosolova, H. A population study of the influence of beer consumption on folate and homocysteine concentrations. Eur J Clin Nutr 2001; 55: 605-609.

31. Ferraro, P. M., Taylor, E. N., Cambaro, G., & Curhan, G. C. Soda and other beverages and the risk of kidney stones. Clin J Am Soc Nephrol 2013; 8: 1389-1395.

32. Romeo. J., Warnberg, J., Nova, E., Diaz, L. E. et al. Changes in the immune system after moderate beer consumption. Ann Nutr Metab 2007; 51: 359-366.

33. Castro-Sepulveda , M., Johannsen, N., Astudillo, S., Jorquera, C. et al. Effects of beer, non-alcoholic beer and water consumption before exercise on fluid and electrolyte homeostasis in athletes. Nutrients 2016; 8: piiE345.

34. Paschall, M., & Lipton, R. I. Wine preference and related health determinants in a U.S national sample of young adults. Drug Alcohol Depend 2005; 78: 339-344.

35. Sluik, D., Brouwer-Brolsma, E. M., de Vries, J. H., Geelen, A. et al. Association of alcoholic beverage preference with cardiometabolic and lifestyle factors: The NQplus study. BMJ Open 2016; 6:010437.

36. Strandberg, T. E., Standberg, A. Y., Salomaa, V. V., Pitkaka. K. et al. Alcoholic beverage preference, 29 year mortality and quality of life in men in old age. J Gerontol A Biol Sci Med Sci 2007;62: 213-218.

37. Kubo, J. T., Stefanick, M. L., Robbins, J., Wactawski-Wende, J., Cullen, M. R. et al. Preference for wine is associated with lower hip fracture incidence in post-menopausal women. BMC Women's Health 2013l 13: 36.

38. Xu, X., Zhu, Y., Zheng, X., & Xie, L. Does beer,

wine or liquor consumption correlate with the risk of renal cell carcinoma? A dose response meta-analysis of prospective cohort studies. Oncotarger 2015; 6: 13347-13358.

39. Sayon-Orea, C., Martinez-Gonzalez, M. A., & Bes-Rastrollo, M. Alcohol consumption and body weight: A systematic review. Nutr Rev 2011; 69: 419-431.

www.ingramcontent.com/pod-product-compliance
Lightning Source LLC
Chambersburg PA
CBHW051429090426
42737CB00014B/2889